"The whole person approach to wellness fits very nicely into the addiction model of recovery, and thus will be a valuable tool within the recovery process."

Merrill Kempfert, Executive Director
Parkside Lutheran Hospital

"Finding a balance between yourself and others is not easy. The Tubesings don't offer a recipe book for achieving that balance, but they do provide helpful resources and principles."

Bookstore Journal

"The Tubesings, experienced psychologists and educators, have offered good advice for everyone caught in the bind of how to strike a healthy balance. Self-tests, provocative questions, and discussion materials make this book suitable for groups or classes."

Medical Self-Care

"Finally—a book which sees the importance of moving beyond wellness and self-care to commitment and service to others. Its underlying theme is that personal well-being requires investment in people and causes beyond oneself."

Granger Westberg
Lutheran General Healthcare System

Whole Person Associates
210 West Michigan
Duluth Minnesota 55802-1908
218-727-0500

Seeking your HEALTHY BALANCE

▶ A Do-it-yourself Guide
to Whole Person Well-being

WORKSHOP IN A BOOK

DONALD A TUBESING & NANCY LOVING TUBESING

Whole Person Associates
210 West Michigan
Duluth Minnesota 55802-1908
218-727-0500

SEEKING YOUR HEALTHY BALANCE
A Do-it-yourself Guide to Whole Person Well-being

This material was originally published in
The Caring Question

Printed in the United States of America by
Edwards Brothers Inc., Ann Arbor MI
10 9 8 7 6 5 4 3

Editorial Director: Susan Gustafson
Assistant Editor: Patrick Gross
Art Director: Joy Morgan Dey
Production Coordinator: Tina P Olson

Library of Congress Cataloging in Publication Data 91-65787
ISBN 0-938586-45-9

To our parents
Dorothy and Butch
Myrt and Karl
who shaped our answers to life's caring questions
and
to our children
Phil and Andy
who have sharpened our understanding
of the healthy balance

Contents

Authors' Preface

The core ideas in this book were originally published by Augsburg Publishing House as **The Caring Question.**

The original **Caring Question** focused on the balance between two issues—self-care and reaching out to others. That dual focus for our caring remains the basic human balance issue with which each of us must struggle. However, in this book we've added work to the balance equation.

The question of how to balance these three major components in our lives is one that, at times, gives even the most capable among us the fits.

In this "workshop in a book" we've asked a lot of questions, and have given you space to formulate your own answers. After all, it's your answers to the caring questions that will ultimately help you find your own healthy balance.

We authors have for years been seeking to maintain our own healthy balance. When necessary, we've struggled to regain it and start over again. We expect to be engaged in this continual rebalancing process for the rest of our lives.

We invite you to continue to seek your healthy balance from among the varied and competing options that your life offers. We hope that the pages to follow will help you in that process.

Donald A. Tubesing/ Nancy Loving Tubesing
6/25/91

1

THE HEALTHY BALANCE

Juggling work, self, and others

Listen to the wellness message of the 90s: To be fully healthy you must take care of yourself—body, mind, and spirit—while at the same time caring for your family, holding a full-time job, and contributing to your community.

Most of us believe that message.

In our current culture we expect to be able to do everything —and to do it well. Men are supposed to be "bread winners," but also gentle friends and fathers, and helpful house-husbands. Women feel the crush between conflicting priorities even more acutely. They're expected to be wives, mothers, and career-oriented professionals—and what's more, they're still supposed to find the time and energy to look like a movie star.

While the concept of a well-balanced life is widely accepted today, attaining it is at least as difficult, if not more difficult, than ever.

- How do you take care of three kids under five and still find time for yourself?
- When do you decide to exercise at noon rather than go to the bank?
- How do you get your studying done when your roommate needs to talk?
- When should you neglect sleep in favor of work?
- How do you attend to your aging parent, as well as your career?
- When should you spend time with friends after work and tell your family to cook their own supper?

Caught between these competing demands for our time and attention, many of us experience distress rather than peace, dis-ease rather than wellness, and we falter and stumble while seeking to keep our balance.

The triple agenda

Earlier generations have emphasized one aspect of balance over the other—focusing on hard work to the neglect of self, or emphasizing personal fulfillment over commitment to family.

Our generation recognizes the importance of self-care, caring for others, and investing in meaningful work. We're encouraged to attend to all aspects of well-being equally. At first glance that seems to be admirable, even healthy.

Self-care. We are bombarded on all fronts with positive self-care messages. Advertisers extol the health benefits of their products. Restaurants offer heart-healthy choices. We cut back on sodium and brag about our cholesterol levels. We engage in low impact aerobic exercise and spend our days in smoke-free workplaces. Ours is a generation with its consciousness raised about wellness behavior.

Admirable and healthy.

Care for others. Our generation is also committed to recapturing the values of family and friendship. We have learned the cost of looking out for self first and have lived through the pain of throw-away relationships. We pride ourselves on being deep, caring people, willing to make a personal sacrifice for others—especially those whom we love.

Admirable and healthy.

Meaningful work. We also look for meaningful work. Just "putting in your time" is no longer in style. Instead we strive to find challenging, stimulating work where we can make a contribution to the wider society in which we live.

Nothing wrong with that.

The common problem of our generation is not that we are ignoring any one major aspect of healthful living—because we aren't. Instead, we're trying so hard to do it all, so well, that we're driving ourselves crazy and making ourselves sick. What a health-eroding trap! The challenge of the 90s is to seek a healthy balance, not to do it all, as if we have no limits.

Consider these examples of typical Americans whose lives are out of balance.

Carol

Carol is in her early forties. She works full time in a responsible job that doesn't pay well, but working conditions are excellent. She often has to work past quitting time to get the job done.

Carol has an active, energetic husband and three teenagers as well. She has obligations to an extended family on both sides. She sings in the church choir and belongs to the Junior League. She's the first one to take in a stray kid or help at the bazaar, but she can barely squeeze in time for a haircut.

This year one of her children had a series of health problems. Carol's bad back bothers her constantly and has stopped her from playing tennis.

Jeff

Jeff just took a new job that he finds incredibly stimulating. He is working long hours and is pouring his heart and soul into learning the ropes.

His family responsibilities are usually tacked onto the end of his day. He sees so little of his children that he is not really a part of their lives. Jeff's marriage and friendships are suffering from neglect. Even his health has been affected since he doesn't sleep well, skips meals, and exercises only when the lawn needs mowing.

Sue

Sue hits the trail at 5 AM every day to get in her first 10-mile run. She continues with yoga before breakfast. In the evening she runs again. She attends an exercise class at the YMCA twice a week and works out on Nautilus the other three days.

Sue's part-time job does not take care of her family's needs but a full-time job would interfere with her training routine. She feels that she has sacrificed for years for her kids. Now it's her turn.

Karl

Karl has graduated from college but can't find a job in his field. He has moved back home to live with his parents. He is working two part-time jobs at the mall and is frustrated by the lack of prospects for his "real" career.

Karl feels tied to his house since his parents still expect him to be home for dinner and in by 11 PM. He struggles with his responsibilities to his parents and his desire for autonomy and space.

Peggy

Peggy is a single parent of two small children. In order to support herself, she works as a secretary. Her boss expects her to be at work on time.

Every morning she bundles up the kids, takes them to day care and rushes to work. Every evening she hurries to pick them up, then races home to make supper. When one of her children is sick she has few alternatives. She has to stay home.

It's been more than a year now since she's had the luxury of asking herself how well she's taking care of herself. The question doesn't even seem relevant.

Choosing your healthy balance

Since our time and energy are, in fact, limited, it's not easy to find the balance between taking care of ourselves, investing in meaningful work, and reaching out to others. Our limits force us to make choices.

Is now the time to take care of me? You? My work? When should I say "no" to you and "yes" to me? When should I help you fulfill yourself, even at cost to me? When must I put my nose to the grindstone, even when I don't feel like it?

- A friend is in crisis and needs your emotional support night after night. How much can you give? For how long?
- You've volunteered to work on the church stewardship drive. How many nights should you work before you take one off to be with yourself and your family?
- You're in the pits. Should you take a mental health day from work even though others will be inconvenienced and your project will be behind schedule?
- You've scheduled a much-needed vacation for yourself but your son has the chance to go to France. Who should get your family's limited travel budget?
- Your boss needs you to work late. Should you cancel your plans or do what you want for yourself?

Dilemmas like this confront us every day—and the choices are tough. How do you find the healthy balance? If you always say "yes" to your outside obligations, you won't be healthy for long. Through plain self-neglect you'll soon wear yourself out in one way or another. If you always say "me first," your life will be shallow and empty. Self-care is not a deep enough purpose for life. Truly healthy people do something with their wellness, even at cost to themselves.

What about you? What does the current balance equation in your life look like? Feel like? Is it healthy for you? The following exercise will help you answer these issues for yourself.

Reflection on Your Current Balance Patterns

- Imagine that the space within the circle below represents all of your available time and energy. Consider the ratio between the amount of your time and attention you currently focus on **self-care**, the amount you focus on **other-care**, and the amount that you focus on **work**. Then divide the circle into three pieces that represent this ratio and label each segment. Of course, you can't be absolutely sure, so just make the best estimate you can of the balance in your life right now.

- Next, using dotted lines, divide your self-care portion into segments that accurately represent your current time and energy investment in the four aspects of self-care: **physical, mental, relational** and **spiritual**. Label each slice.

- In the same way divide the **other-care** portion to reflect your present time investment in **family, friends** and **reaching out** to others in your community. Label each section.

- Finally, divide the **work** section of your circle to represent your current investment in your **job** and **service to causes** that are important to you. Label the slices appropriately.

  Note: If you don't have any idea how you're spending your time and energy these days, keep track of your activities for a week; then come back and complete this exercise.

Consider your investment in self-care, other-care, and in work.

■ What is your primary commitment in self-care (the biggest slice of the self-care segment)?

_____

■ What is your primary commitment in other-care (the biggest slice of the other-care segment)?

_____

■ What is your primary commitment to meaningful work and causes?

_____

■ How do you feel about your healthy balance as represented by your overall division of this circle? Will this balance be sustaining for you over the long run?

_____

_____

■ How does this picture fit with your personal values and priorities?

_____

_____

■ Would you like to adjust your time and energy spending patterns in any way?

_____

■ Would you like to increase the size of any investments? Which ones?

_____

■ Which slice or slices would you be willing to reduce to reinvest more time in your other priorities? _____

Don't cheat here! Be honest. When you increase your commitment in one area, you'll have to decrease it in another. If you'd like to add in something new, but you're unwilling to cut anything out, you're not only fooling yourself, but also setting yourself up for failure.

The healthy balance dilemma

In our "super person" society, you're supposed to take care of yourself, as well as everyone else, to find a satisfying job that keeps your body and soul (not to mention your family!) together, and still find time for volunteering!

Does that message sound familiar?

"How do I successfully juggle all that?" you ask.

Unfortunately, there are no easy formulas for how you can commit yourself to permanent relationships and work-related responsibilities, and still remain responsive to your own ever-changing feelings and needs.

This book is intended to help you look at the ways in which you are currently investing yourself in these various responsibilities as you search to find your healthy balance. It will also provide you with some options you may not have actively considered as you explore the healthy balance issues, one at a time:

- You can't be well without taking care of yourself.
  (Chapters 2–7)
- You can't be well without investing in meaningful work and reaching out to others.
  (Chapters 8–11)
- Finding a healthy balance is an on-going process.
  (Chapters 12 and 13)

Remember, it's your life, your energy, and your time. You must decide where to invest it—where to invest yourself!

No one else can decide for you. You alone can chart your course and make your investments and commitments. Even if you think that someone else is deciding for you, they're not! You're just giving them permission to do so for you, and **that's your choice**!

So, the challenge is, in light of your values and beliefs, to invest yourself where it counts—to invest yourself in a balance between self-care, other-care, and meaningful work that you believe in, that you can live with and be proud of, and that ultimately you will be willing to die with as your legacy. Invest yourself so that you can look back on your life and say that in your own way you did what you could to make the world a better place.

How do you find that healthy balance?

You've already made a start by picking up this book. Surely you had a number of other responsibilities crying for your attention.

The next step is to look at the major principles of positive self-care.

2

KEEPING BODY and SOUL TOGETHER

Creative self-care

Most people are interested in their health. They generally become concerned about it, however, only when some symptom forces them to pay attention—a runny nose, a pain in the chest, an ankle sprain, insomnia, weight gain. Most of us take health for granted until troublesome symptoms "prove" to us that we are "sick" or "disabled." Then, forced to notice, we pay attention and react to correct the problem. The most effective self-care, however, results from a conscious decision to take care of yourself before you get sick.

How do you go about taking care of yourself? This chapter will explore four main ideas that form a foundation for effective self-care:

- Health is wholeness.
- Health requires personal responsibility.
- Health represents a return on your investment.
- Health requires self-nurture.

Health is wholeness

Health is more than having a body that works. Health includes the physical, emotional, intellectual, social, and spiritual dimensions of life, which when working in harmony, lead to a sense of well-being and satisfaction.

The question on a job application that asks you to check whether your health is "good," "fair," or "poor" usually refers to the state of your body. Yet both the job applicant and the personnel manager know that physical health is profoundly affected by emotions, relationships, and lifestyle.

Although we usually think about health in physical terms, it really involves all of you—your mind, your connections with people, your sense of hope, your emotions, your satisfaction with work—as well as your body. Health is a multifaceted subject.

Really, we are one single system, a whole. We use many different words to describe sickness and well-being within the components of our life—physical, emotional, social, intellectual, and spiritual. But these distinctions are really verbal fiction. There aren't different forms of sickness or of health. In reality, sickness is a disruption of wholeness in whatever form it occurs, and healing is a return to wholeness by whatever means.

There is a unity to the nature of brokenness in its many forms (whether torn ligaments, ruptured vessels, bone fractures, split personalities, broken hearts, or lives gone to pieces). And there is a unity to the nature of healing in its variety of forms that brings wholeness and new life.

We struggle for wholeness and personal unity against whatever forces tend to wound us, and we heal naturally, by grace, through the process of living:

- Our bodies self-correct through internal regulation (homeostasis).
- Our emotions seek peace and acceptance in the face of worry.
- Our intellect uses logic and memory to counteract confusion.
- We respond to our social environment by making up, giving in, speaking up, or fighting back.
- In the face of despair our spirits seek hope, faith, and meaning.

We are always in the process of struggling for an experience of life that tells us with a rush of energy that we are again whole. The synergy of wholeness generates the tingling sense of being fully alive.

To be truly effective, self-care must take seriously our behaviors in every facet of living and not focus only on physical

15

self-care. All of our lifestyle habits should be examined and judged by whether they create disintegration or wholeness.

Health requires personal responsibility

Self-care is essential. What you do to and for yourself makes a great deal of difference. Take care of your body, your mind, your relationships, and your spirit, and they will return to you a measure of health. Ignore them, or worse, engage in self-destructive habits, and you will soon pay the price. Take physical health as an example.

Physical health over the life span is as much a result of personal lifestyle and health habits as it is a matter of good fortune. We're not just victims of bad luck. God does not give heart disease; it's man-made—and now woman-made too! In our country, today, more people die from overeating than from malnutrition.

It's our own fault. If we've learned anything in health care in the last few years, it's that health doesn't just happen. And sickness doesn't just leap from the woods and grab us; we grow it in our own gardens. Two epidemic killers of our generation, heart disease and stroke, are not the result of fate, an ill wind, or a bug. They are related to lifestyle. We seldom catch our death of anything anymore; we get it the old-fashioned way—we earn it!

All too often we treat ourselves as we treat our cars—mechanically. If nothing is wrong with a car, it's "healthy." If it's not working right, it's "sick." We tend to drive our cars as fast and as far as possible until something breaks. Then we haul it into a shop and say, "fix it." When it's repaired, we get it back on the road and drive it as fast and as far as possible again.

So also with ourselves. All too often being healthy simply means, "I am in working order, and I can go about my daily business accomplishing as much as I can as quickly as possible. When something does go wrong, and I can't go on any longer, I haul myself in, shouting, 'Fix me, and get me back on the road as soon as possible so I can drive myself like crazy again.'" Not a very effective long-range plan for either cars or people!

This physical health principle is just as true for other aspects of personal self-care. If you want your mind to remain as open and alive at 70 as it was at 20, you'll have to exercise it, encourage its curiosity, and provide it with regular stimulation and challenge. Relationships not cultivated soon wither. They thrive on contact and mutual sharing and support. A spirit undernourished turns cynical and dies. Your spirit needs daily attention. For your whole person to remain vital, you'll have to take responsibility for nourishing all aspects of your health—body, mind, and spirit.

Health represents a return on your investment

Maximum long-term health is most likely to be found in individuals who choose to invest their energies in a health-enhancing life-style. Health-producing habits are the world's best medicine.

Most working people regularly pay into a pension plan designed to provide financial security in retirement years. The amount that's put into the plan each day is very small, but over the years it adds up.

Everyone contributes regularly to a health pension plan. The long-range investments you make in your health accumulate over the years. Viewed on a day-to-day basis, your investment in a nap after lunch, a stretch break at work, a phone call to a friend, or a five-minute break to watch the sunset doesn't seem to have much long-term effect on your health. That extra cup of coffee, one more rushed hour, another angry argument, or a cynical remark don't seem as if they should detract from your health 20 years from now. But they do. These little bits do add up over the long run.

It's not just the major tragedies and traumas of life that determine your health in the future. Most of those you can't control anyway, so why focus on them? It's the small habits, the daily decisions (just one more cigar, one more time-pressured job, one more deception, one more short night's sleep) that accumulate in your future-health account. Health and sickness are to a large extent the result of daily choices, repeated over the years, to do for ourselves small favors or disfavors.

What about your health investment plan? Think about your choices today. Have you been saving for health or disease? Will your day full of seemingly insignificant behaviors contribute over the long run to wearing you out, or have you been making long-range investments in your future health? Multiplied 10,000 times over the next 30 years, which of your self-care habits would contribute to your health and which would lead toward illness?

Check out your Health Portfolio using the following worksheet.

Health Investment Portfolio

■ What little favors have you done for yourself today that will add up to positive self-care habits and long-range investments in your health? (Examples: eating a leisurely balanced breakfast, walking to work, making an affirming phone call, taking three deep breaths.)

_____

_____

Multiplied 10,000 times over the next 30 years, these activities will help immensely in moving you toward your health-investment goals.

■ Now the other side of the balance sheet. What insults have you offered yourself today that are long-range investments in a future disabling illness? (Examples: three cups of coffee, rushing to meet the bus, shouting at the kids, beer and potato chips at the game.)

_____

_____

Multiplied 10,000 times over the next 30 years, these and other negative self-care habits will probably kill you before your time!

■ Are there any changes you would like to make? _____

_____

_____

Health requires self-nurture

To foster positive self-care habits you must be willing to care-fully nurture yourself. You need to cultivate an "I'm worth it" attitude.

Many people are so busy paying attention to the demands of work and the needs of others that they rarely stop long enough to give to themselves. They end up so focused on others that to them self-nurture is a foreign, even threatening idea.

Whole person wellness doesn't advocate abandonment of the ideals of service and sacrifice in favor of self-indulgence. The fact remains, however, that self-care is essential for good health.

Even though self-care may feel awkward and faintly sacrilegious, it's certainly the appropriate starting point for promoting your own vitality. What would it mean for you to nurture yourself? Feed yourself? Pamper yourself? Take care of yourself? Stand up for yourself?

The suggestions below will give you some starters. The next chapters will offer many more. But remember, in personal self-care lack of information is usually not the problem. Good ideas are not enough. Good intentions are not sufficient either. You must be willing to care-fully care for yourself. And that requires action on your part!

Three steps to self-care

Listen to yourself and learn what fills you. Listening is a gift. You give it to others, you can also give it to yourself. Do you know what fills you? Nurtures you? Feeds you? Listen to your pulse, your feet, your shoulders. Listen to your hopes and your spirit. Listen to your sadness and your joy. If you're hungry for a pizza, a glass of water won't be as satisfying. If you're hungry for love, shopping probably won't help. If your body is exhausted for lack of exercise, napping isn't the treatment it needs. Listen to yourself. You may need excitement, freedom, laughter, tenderness, or serenity.

You could give yourself a lecture or a pat on the back. You could pamper yourself with a gift or a massage. You could go to a movie, read a book or take a bubble bath. But you can't fill yourself until you know what you need. Ask yourself, "Given all the circumstances in my life right now, what would it mean for me to take better care of myself?" Listen to your answer. Then:

Take action to care for yourself. Do something for yourself that fills a need. Don't wait for a miracle or a knight in shining armor. Don't wait for "them"—whoever they are—to notice your need. Stoke your fires yourself, and rekindle your own spirit.

Set aside time each day for yourself. Schedule a regular self-care time, even if you start with only five minutes. The regular time will help you keep yourself on your own list of needy people and will help you focus. You have the right to take care of yourself. Give yourself permission to do so!

Evaluate your habits

The next four chapters outline specific self-care strategies for promoting physical, mental, relational, and spiritual health. But before you read on, please stop and reflect for a moment about your current self-care habits. How well do you take care of yourself in each of the dimensions of life?

The inventory below will give you some idea of your current self-care patterns. You may be surprised by some of the questions. "What does laughter have to do with health?" you may ask. What about forgiveness? Seat belts? Or friendships? You'll get to all these issues in later chapters. For now, go ahead and check the statements that apply to you.

Whole Person Health Habit Inventory

Physical

__ I participate regularly (three times a week or more) in a vigorous physical-exercise program.

__ I eat a well-balanced diet.

__ My weight is within 10 lbs. of the ideal weight for my height.

__ My alcohol consumption is seven drinks (shot, beer, or glass of wine) or fewer per week.

__ I always wear my seat belt.

__ I do not smoke cigarettes, cigars or a pipe.

__ I generally get adequate and satisfying sleep.

Mental

__ I seldom experience periods of depression.

__ I generally face up to problems and cope with change effectively.

__ I worry very little about future possibilities or things I can't change.

__ I laugh several times a day and usually fit "play" into my schedule.

__ I am curious and always on the lookout for new learning.

__ I maintain a realistic and basically positive self-image.

__ I choose to feel confident and optimistic.

Relational

__ I seek help and support when I need it.

__ I have at least one friend with whom I can share almost anything.

__ I have nourishing intimate relationships with family and/or friends.

__ I experience and express a wide range of emotions and respond to others' feelings appropriately.

__ Each day includes comfortable and stimulating interaction with others.

__ I solicit and accept feedback from others.

__ I stick up for myself when it's necessary and appropriate.

Spiritual

__ I set aside 15-20 minutes each day for prayer or meditation.

__ I participate in regular spiritual rituals with people who share my beliefs.

__ I accept my limitations and inadequacies without embarrassment or apology.

__ I keep the purpose of my life clearly in mind and let it guide my goal setting and decision making.

__ I regularly offer my time and possessions in service to others.

__ I am sensitive to ultimate truths and the spiritual dimension of life.

__ I readily forgive myself and others.

Count up your check marks for each category and record them below.

Physical _____   Relational _____

Mental _____   Spiritual _____   TOTAL _____

- How to interpret your score:

The total number of checks on the **Whole Person Health Habit Inventory** provides a general idea of how well you take care of your health across all dimensions of life. Compare your total score to the healthy balance standards:

24-28 Excellent: Your habits are enhancing your health.

16-23 Average: You're obviously trying, but there's room for improvement.

Below 16 Poor: The quality of your health is probably diminished by your poor habits.

Take a few minutes to reflect on your score and your reactions to it. Use the worksheet below to record your insights and resolutions for change.

Personal Reflection on My Self-Care Patterns

- In which areas are my habits an asset? _____

_____

- In which areas are my habits a liability? _____

_____

- In which areas would I like to make changes? _____

_____

- Which particular habits would I like to modify? _____

_____

_____

Take the next step

For specifics on your self-care style, pay particular attention to your score in each of the four categories: physical, mental, relational, spiritual. If you checked three or fewer items in any dimension, you're neglecting your health in that area. If you aren't yet experiencing symptoms, you probably soon will. Be sure to read the appropriate self-care chapter and take action to modify your habits.

In those areas where you checked four or five items, you're probably taking adequate care of yourself. Your self-care habits do enhance your health, but you might consider upgrading some for optimal well-being. There's still room for improvement. Check the corresponding self-care chapter for some new strategies.

Positive responses to six or seven questions in any category indicate that you are practicing positive self-care habits. Congratulations! Over the long run your choices will enhance the quality of your life and your health, and will help you achieve a healthy balance in all dimensions.

As you explore your health habit patterns in the next four chapters, rejoice where you've done well and zero in on those aspects of health where you need to boost your self-care investment.

3

BUILDING a HEALTHY BODY

Physical self-care

Dear Warren,

It's about time you noticed! So glad my headache finally got to you. I was beginning to think I'd have to zap you with a heart attack before you'd pay attention. Just because I'm not very demanding, that doesn't mean I don't have need—like sleep. You seem to think my energy reserves are limitless. Better think again. Unless you slow down, I'm going to break down. Do you read me?

Over and out,

Your Body

Dear Chris,

How long has it been since you checked me? Once a month would be appropriate. Breast cancer is the leading cause of death for women in your age group, and early detection usually is lifesaving. I know you were brought up not to "touch" yourself, but this is really important. You're such a caring, giving person. I'd hate to see your life of love and service cut short.

With concern,

Your Torso

Dear Dan,

Ouch! What are you doing to me? Why do I have to carry all your problems around for you? Please let me put them down once in a while.

Your Aching Back

Dear Sally,

The stretching you've been doing is super! I really appreciate it! I'm also delighted you've stopped trying to beat Alice's pace in the pool. You were pushing me too hard for a while. Just because exercise is good for me doesn't mean that *more* or *harder* exercise is better.

Thanks for listening,

Your Body

Dear George,

Do me a favor, please. Keep track for the next month of all the booze you drink. Every drop. Then come back with a plan for changing that, before I'm totally incapacitated.

Sincerely,

Your Liver

How about you? How does your body feel about how you've been treating it lately? If your body could write you a letter, what would it say?

Physical Self-Care Report Card

- Stop for a minute and grade yourself on the way you've taken care of your body this past week. Give yourself a separate grade for both effort and achievement.

	Effort	Achievement
What I've put into my body (eating, drinking, smoking)	_____	_____
What I've done to it (pace, workload, pressure)	_____	_____
What I've done with it (exercise)	_____	_____
How I've let it rest (sleep, relaxation)	_____	_____

- In what areas would you like to improve your grade for the next week?

_____

Wake up to your body

As we were growing up, most of us took our physical health for granted. Unless we had physical limitations or we became sick and couldn't go on, we never thought much about our health. Our parents took responsibility for trying to ensure a relatively healthy diet and sleep pattern. They may even have insisted on regular exercise. They took us in for checkups, made sure our immunizations were up to date, kissed our minor pains away, and worried when appetites waned or cheeks flushed.

Many of us who absorbed these physical health-care principles into our lifestyle never consciously accepted responsibility for our own health promotion. We more likely shifted the responsibility to a spouse, to our physician, or to fate. Some of us who learned good self-care health habits don't practice what we know. We smoke. We drink. We eat too much of the wrong things. We experiment with drugs. We're careless about safety precautions. We're too busy to exercise. We don't pay attention to early warning signals. Or we spend too much time worrying about every twinge and ache.

As long as our lives are free from pain or disease and as long as we are able to function as we wish and have adequate energy, we are not likely to worry too much about our physical health. We start paying attention when our bodies let us down. You get mono or herpes. You slip a disc or break your wrist. Your hay fever blossoms. Your appendix ruptures. A physical exam reveals hypertension or a hernia. Your cramps seem unbearable. That nagging headache won't go away. You can't sleep. A motorcycle accident lands you in the hospital with a crushed hip. Toxic shock syndrome threatens your life and your childbearing.

Suddenly physical well-being becomes an important issue for you, perhaps a life-and-death issue. When your body writes nasty, painful letters, you're more inclined to take the message seriously. Whether it occurs through illness or accident or a health class, this kind of awareness usually marks the beginning of responsible self-care.

Build self-care habits

Health care is something you do every day. It's easy to take your body for granted and not realize you are paying a price. What you do for yourself over the years has a tremendous impact on how you feel physically and how you feel about yourself.

Up to about 25 years of age your body increases in energy and strength. It's remarkable the amount of reserve a

20-year-old body has in the bank. From about 25 on you start a long slide, as your energy reserves and strength decline. But you don't notice it right away. Somewhere in the middle or late 40s, people suddenly realize that they are increasingly becoming a maintenance problem. It's then that the results of your self-care habits over the years start to show clearly.

Ours is the first generation possessing the knowledge and technology that enables us to deliberately increase our life span by making healthy choices. We know that buckling up for safety as we drive can increase the odds for adding years to our life. We're bombarded with information about the life-shortening effects of smoking cigarettes. We know that if we exercise regularly and scrutinize our diets we can minimize the risk of strokes and heart attacks.

We may even receive a computer printout of our health risks and life expectancy along with an annual physical exam. Long life is certainly one goal of physical health care. Quality of life is another. We all want to die as old as possible, feeling as young as possible, perhaps with as little pain as possible.

Physical well-being is also important to us in the short run. You could characterize well-being as having the capacity to function as you wish, adequate energy to go through your day without physical fatigue, strength to meet the challenges you encounter, and endurance to maintain your desired pace. Your standards for well-being may differ greatly from your neighbor's: she may need the strength to climb a telephone pole, while you need only carry a briefcase.

When it comes right down to it, the specifics of a physical self-care plan are highly personal. It's your body and your life. You know what you want from and for yourself and what you're willing to invest or sacrifice.

There are four major areas that you ought to consider in your physical self-care plan: exercise, relaxation, nutrition, and the use of chemicals. Each area has both long and short-range costs and benefits in relation to personal limitations, energy, strength, and endurance.

Exercise: build your stamina

Americans are exercising in ever-increasing numbers. Designer running shoes and exercise clothes have become the status symbols of the 90s. People exercise for weight control, for strength, for endurance, for cardiovascular fitness, for the camaraderie and challenge of a sport, for peace of mind, and to keep up with the Joneses. Most of us know that "exercise is good for you" but are only vaguely aware of "how much" or "which kind" or "for what purpose."

Physical fitness experts suggest that all of us should be able to lift our own body weight using only our arms and shoulders. If you can't do a chin-up, exercises to strengthen your upper body would seem appropriate. If a trim physical appearance is important to your sense of well-being, calisthenics and tummy tighteners are in order.

However, if maximum well-being is your goal, aerobic exercise is the choice. Moderate exercise (just twenty minutes at a time) on a regular basis (three times a week) will help you increase the capacity of your lungs, strengthen your heart, and develop muscular efficiency. This development of your heart-lung capacity (called cardiovascular fitness) improves circulation so that your body receives more nutrients and oxygen while efficiently ridding itself of wastes. Your enzyme system stays balanced, your muscles can relax more completely, you fall asleep more easily, and your endurance increases.

People who exercise regularly report other benefits, including good muscle tone, a general feeling of well-being, relief from depression, tension release, and weight control. Paradoxical as it sounds, you will probably have far more energy following exercise than you did before. Our bodies seem to thrive on regular exercise. When you feel down and tired, you may need to exercise rather than to relax.

What about you? How do you feel about your current level of physical activity?

Physical Activity Assessment

- Are you exercising on a regular basis? Why? Why not? _____

_____

- Does your routine include aerobic conditioning? _____

- Do you have any limitations that prevent regular exercise? _____

_____

- What changes in your exercise habits might enhance your well-being? _____

_____

If you'd like to modify your exercise patterns, here are seven strategies for building your stamina. They will be useful in providing you with a common sense way of getting started.

Seven stamina builders

Check your attitude. Ask yourself whether you are willing to exercise at least every other day. If you're not, then you should not exercise at all. Irregular exertion for which your body isn't prepared does more harm than good. There's truth in the old joke: if you want to know when you will die, be a weekend athlete—you'll probably die on a weekend.

Design an aerobic program that makes sense for you. Almost any exercise that makes your heart work hard will suffice: walking, swimming, cross-country skiing, tennis, jumping rope, climbing stairs, calisthenics, dancing, bicycling. Do what you most enjoy. The key is steady exercise that keeps your heartbeat elevated for at least twenty minutes three times a week.

Start slowly and build gradually. Don't push yourself too hard. Increase your capacity over a year, not over a week or two. Know your own limits. Start by stretching and exercising lightly. Then don't push yourself too hard, even after you're fit. If you feel tired rather than energized one hour after exertion, then you've probably done too much. Cut back for a while. If you're training to be healthy, exercise should never hurt.

Always warm up and cool down. Spend five minutes warming up before exercising and five minutes cooling down afterwards. Give your body a chance to get ready for the pace and to recover from the exertion. It's tempting to skip these steps when you're pressed for time. Don't give in! That's when you need the transition most. Systematically stretch each muscle every day. We're only beginning to learn the importance of stretching both as an adjunct to exercise and as an intrinsically healthy activity.

Build supports and rewards into your program. Start an exercise chart with daily gold stars and periodic rewards for persistence. Treat yourself to a movie after a week or a new swimsuit after a month. Notch your miles on a walking stick or a pedometer. Add music to your routine. Exercising with friends or family may provide mutual encouragement as well as relief from boredom. If you don't like exercising alone, find ways to combat the loneliness of the long-distance runner.

Combine exercise goals. If looking fit and trim is important to you, add exercises to tone and shape the body (sit-ups, push-ups, leg lifts, weights) to your aerobic routine. Yoga postures provide physical conditioning that helps maintain flexibility and decrease muscular tension.

Exercise up to your limitations. With an ounce of precaution and a pound of creativity, those of us with physical limitations can devise an aerobic exercise program. If you are over 35 or have any serious illness, especially heart problems, consult your physician before exercising. Walking may be the best starting point for you, and it's an excellent exercise for anyone.

When you exercise regularly, you'll look and feel better and will be able to ward off the negative effects of distress more effectively. After you're into it, regular exercise acts as a stimulant. It's a healthy high, a positive addiction. Physical fitness may not add years to your life, but it will add life to your years. Prevent rust and rot—exercise!

A note to non-believers

If your exercise these days has been limited to climbing walls, dragging your heels, flying off the handle, or running around in circles, you're probably feeling guilty with all this focus on aerobics. Good! Keep on feeling that way until it's so uncomfortable that you do something about it. Then come back to this chapter and plan an exercise program that meets your needs and fits your lifestyle. Exercise fanatics can be tough to live with. When you do decide to start exercising, choose an activity and pace that's right for you, and avoid making comparisons.

Relaxation: short-circuit the stress connection

Stress is one of the most pervasive and intriguing health problems of our times. The stress response is a marvelous mind/body mechanism that gears us up to meet dangerous situations with an extra burst of energy.

Unfortunately, we tend to abuse this energy resource by calling on it too often—overloading our schedules, overreacting to people and life events, overburdening ourselves with worries or expectations. Some of us run the danger flag up too often. It's as if we shift into passing gear to get out of a tight spot and then have trouble gearing down.

When we push ourselves at high speed all the time, we're likely to run out of gas more quickly, and lose our emergency acceleration power.

Stress seems to have a similar effect on our bodies. Many of us suffer the side effects of chronic stress—unresolved muscle tension, elevated blood pressure, increased heartbeat, general arousal. We don't know how to get out of passing gear. Eventually the tension, arousal, and tightness seem normal, and we find ourselves more vulnerable to illness and poor self-care habits. Chronic tension can knot muscles, lower mobility, degenerate joints, cause spine problems, and exhaust us.

Systematic relaxation reverses the emergency stress response by decreasing unconscious muscular tension and regulating breathing. Since most people don't really know how to relax, the process takes practice and persistence.

You can relax in a hundred different ways. Each method is, of course, somewhat different from the others, but each is based on the same principle. By exercising your powers of consciousness, you can modify most, if not all, of your physiological processes, including your heartbeat and blood pressure. By using any of the popular relaxation methods, you can learn to release tension and thereby control your stress.

What about you? Have you found effective ways to relax?

Relaxation Assessment

■ In what ways do you normally relax? _____

■ How often and when? _____

■ Is your present style efficient and effective for you? _____

■ What recommendation would you make to yourself about even more healthy patterns?

_____

_____

If you choose tension-reduction as one of your routes to fuller health, the five roads to relaxation described below will give you some direction. Remember, for relaxation to help, you must do it. Knowing that you could relax if you wanted to won't get you the results you need. Self-care for chronic tension begins with letting go. Make deep relaxation one of your daily habits!

Five roads to relaxation

Use any one method of relaxation each day for one month. Practice the approach you select for at least 20 minutes each day. At the end of the month evaluate the impact of your program on your sense of well-being and vitality.

Systematically check your physical tension level. Then consciously relax the muscles where you find tension. Here's how. Stretch each muscle, then release the tension. Notice which muscles you have been holding tight. Test your whole body, one part at a time. Check your hands, wrists, forearms, upper arms, shoulders, neck, face, jaw, chest, back, groin, stomach, thighs, calves, ankles, feet, and toes. Where do you hold tension? Once you're aware of your favorite storage places, you can check your tension level throughout the day by focusing on these spots.

Periodically relax your favorite tension spots. To relax a particular tension area, tighten the muscles, then let go fully; repeat three times. Or imagine, as you breathe in, that you're inflating the tight muscle; when you breathe out, imagine the muscle deflating until you can feel your pulse in it.

Take "yawn and belly-breathing breaks"—at least three every hour. Stand and stretch, then open your mouth and the back of your throat. Stretch until a yawn catches and carries you for a moment. If you're too tight, you can't yawn. Keep at this until you can yawn. A yawn creates total tension, then complete relaxation. It's effective, and it feels good.

Clear your mind and prepare for sleep. Focus on relaxing at the end of each day. Don't rehash the whole day's troubles right up until bedtime. You need some time away from the pressure. If you've struggled with a problem all day, at night you need to let go. Give up the problems of the day and let go! The key is that you must be willing to slack off.

Sometimes a long walk or vigorous exercise helps. Giving or receiving a massage, taking a warm bath, and drinking a glass of milk at bedtime can all be effective late-evening relaxants.

Develop the expectation that sleep will allow peace and strength to creep back into your pores and joints. Envision this healing action taking place.

Nutrition:
build strong bodies

Eating is a daily process of finding your healthy balance of essential nutrients and caloric intake. Nutritional self-care focuses on two habit patterns—what you eat (the content) and how you eat (the process). Take a look at the content of your diet first.

Nutrition Assessment

- Think back to yesterday and see if you can remember everything you ingested during the day:

  breakfast _____, _____, _____, _____, _____

  coffee break _____, _____, _____

  lunch _____, _____, _____, _____, _____

  after-school snack _____, _____, _____

  after-work cocktails _____, _____, _____

  supper _____, _____, _____, _____, _____

  late-night snacks _____, _____, _____

  a nightcap _____, _____, _____

- How many calories would you estimate you took in yesterday? _____

Check the labels on the food you eat, and add up the calories you typically consume.

In the first half of life men generally need 2,500–3,000 calories per day, depending on their physical activity levels. Women require about 2,000 calories. After you're 45 years old this number begins to drop by about 100 calories per decade.

If you take in more than you need, and maintain that pattern, you'll gain weight unless you exercise to expend the extra calories. If you take in less than you need, and maintain that pattern, you'll lose weight. You'll lose more if you also exercise. That's all there is to weight control. If you're within 10 pounds of the recommended standard weight for your height, your calorie intake is probably just about right.

But healthy nutrition means more than weight control. Food is more than calories. We eat not only to satisfy our hunger, but also to provide our body with the nutrients it needs to maintain well-being. Our body needs fuel (proteins) to repair itself and regulators (vitamins, minerals, and fiber) to keep our systems in balance.

Go back to your list of calories for yesterday. How much of what you ate was empty calories (sugar, junk food, alcohol, soda)? If the percentage is over 10, you're flirting with danger in the long run. The remaining 90 percent (or 60 or 50 percent) of your calories has to provide all of the 55 nutrients your body needs to stay healthy. No wonder Orson Welles quipped, "One-third of what we eat keeps us alive. The other two-thirds keeps our doctors alive!"

Six of the ten leading causes of death in the United States have been linked to diet. It makes good sense to develop our eating skills so that we can make smart choices.

Although nutrition may seem complicated, you don't need to be a chemist or dietitian to improve your eating patterns. Mostly you need common sense, and a few basic principles.

Four food fundamentals

Keep your weight normal. Be calorie wise. Eat only as much food as your body uses. Cut down on portion sizes rather than cutting out food. Remember, calories in alcohol count too! One drink (100 calories) is five percent of a 2000 calorie diet.

Cut down on sugar and sweets. Sugar accounts for one-fourth of the calories in most Americans' diets. Corn syrup, fructose, dextrose, raw sugar, brown sugar, and turbinado sugar are all still sugar! Sugar calories slide down too easily, too quickly—up to 600 calories per minute.

Eat less fat and cholesterol. All kinds of fats seem to lead to heart disease. Choose lean cuts; trim fat before cooking; bake, broil, or boil. Avoid prepared meats; substitute legumes; avoid spreads and dressings. Cut out rich desserts. Use low-fat milk products.

Reduce salt intake. Excess salt has been linked to high blood pressure. Season creatively with lemon, onion, garlic, wine, herbs, spices. Convenience foods are loaded with salt and other sodium compounds. Avoid processed foods. Cut recipe portion of salt to one-half or less.

Change eating habits

Eating satisfies a variety of needs in addition to physical hunger. When do you eat? Why do you eat? How do you eat? These questions invite you to reflect on the process of eating and the complicated array of emotional rewards most of us connect with our food.

Eating is one of the primary ways we receive nurturing. When you were very small, you probably got lots of warmth and cuddling and love talk and affirmation along with the milk. Some of us still look forward to mealtime as an opportunity to fill ourselves up emotionally as well as physically. That can cause problems!

It's also likely that some lifelong eating habits got started when you were a youngster. Did you dawdle around at feeding time or gulp and run? Were you deprived of food when you were hungry or forced to eat more than you desired? Were mealtimes intimate moments in your family or arenas for conflict?

Eating Habits Inventory

■ Stop for a minute and take an inventory of your eating habits from the process viewpoint.

	Usually	Sometimes	Never
Do you tend to eat in response to anxiety, tension, depression?	____	____	____
Do you eat at the same time as you participate in other activities, such as reading, watching TV, cooking?	____	____	____
Do you use eating as your primary mode of celebration?	____	____	____
Do you eat when you're not really hungry?	____	____	____
Do you eat quickly from the beginning of the meal to the end?	____	____	____
Is a clean plate, rather than a full feeling, your cue that you are done eating?	____	____	____
Are you easily stimulated to eat by TV advertisements, billboards, magazine pictures?	____	____	____
Do you enjoy discussing food?	____	____	____
Do you feel compelled to eat food that is offered by others so they won't be offended?	____	____	____
Do you binge and then feel guilty?	____	____	____

43

If you answered usually to more than one of these questions, you may be using food in an addictive pattern. Overeating is a learned addiction. You're probably more sensitive to the smell of food and to TV ads. Foodaholics eat when they're hungry—and when they're tired, bored, angry, depressed, celebrating, or socializing.

If eating satisfies more than physical hunger for you, your self-care habits will need to include learning how to identify your hungers and how to satisfy at least some of them with other kinds of nourishment—like stimulation or laughter or enriching conversation.

What about you? How do you feel about the way you nurture your body and about your eating style? Is there anything you would like to change in order to enhance your well-being?

Before leaving the issue of physical self-care, especially as it relates to nutrition and nurture, we need to take a look at one other area of health habits: the use of alcohol, drugs, and other substances that can have a dramatic, sometimes devastating effect on our minds and bodies.

Chemical use:
the hidden costs of chemicals

Have you used any drugs today? No?

What about caffeine (in cola, coffee, tea, cocoa, chocolate)? Tobacco? Over-the-counter or prescription drugs? Marijuana? Alcohol?

We are a "feel-good" society. Bombarded with messages that tell us we should not be tired, tense, depressed, or in pain, we turn to chemicals, stimulants, and drugs to escape that pain. Covering up our discomfort can be a costly choice. When we override our personal biofeedback mechanism, we lose touch with our own internal wisdom about well-being and we short-circuit our early-warning system.

Smoking is another expensive pleasure. The price is emphysema, chronic bronchitis, lung cancer, heart disease. Not now, maybe not five years from now, but someday you'll pay the price. Tobacco companies have spent billions of dollars trying to link smoking to the beautiful, sexy things in life. In real life smoking is linked only to disability and death.

The use of chemicals, just like food, can be addicting. Caffeine is the most widely used mood-altering drug in America. Do your six cups of coffee or four Diet Cokes a day represent an addiction? Research indicates that an ounce of alcohol daily may be health-full. Is your wine before bed or beer after work relaxing or addicting? Or both? Alcohol is still the most abused drug in our culture. Valium is the most overprescribed.

Chemical Use Assessment

- Which chemicals do you use regularly? _____

- How do you feel about this quantity and pattern of use?_____

- How does your use and/or abuse of chemicals affect your overall health? _____

  _____

  _____

- What positive effect would you expect if you changed that pattern?_____

  _____

You alone know whether you should slow down or stop your use of one or a number of these substances.

Promote fan mail

Careful attention to the four areas of physical self-care—exercise, relaxation, nutrition, and chemical use—will allow your body to give you the energy you need to do the things you want in life for yourself and for others. Want to receive a love letter from your body? Give it the care you would give a lover. Love it gently. Love it daily.

Dear Self,

Thanks for listening to my needs!

Love, Your Body

Before moving on to consider mental self-care, please stop and reflect on your overall physical self-care habits. Do they enhance or erode your well-being?

Personal Reflection on My Physical Health

■ My exercise patterns (type of exercise, regularity, intensity, current physical condition)

_____

_____

■ My relaxation patterns (stress, methods, preparation for sleep) _____

_____

_____

■ My eating patterns (weight, nutrition, eating style) _____

_____

_____

■ My chemical-use patterns (caffeine, alcohol, smoking, other) _____

_____

Wish List for My Physical Health

■ List here everything you can imagine wanting for your physical health-fullness. What would you like to be able to do? To know? To feel? To stop? Let your imagination run free. Don't limit yourself in any way. The wishes don't have to be practical. Have fun dreaming.

I wish I could: _____

_____

_____

_____

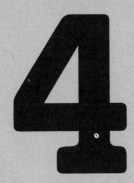

A BETTER IDEA
Mental self-care

From the healthy balance perspective, the second natural focus for self-care is mental health-fullness. Unfortunately, the term mental health all too often has a bad name in our culture, calling up images of craziness, behavioral problems, and emotional outbursts.

The medical profession has tried to help us understand the mind-body connection, but the label psychosomatic (mind-body) illness is all too frequently interpreted as a putdown, a judgment of weakness rather than an affirmation of the miraculous mystery and powerful potential of our minds. Too bad we don't talk more often about psychosomatic health!

What is mental health?

Mental health is more than "nerves" or avoiding "the crazies" or illness that's "all in your head" or a "figment of your imagination." Mental health encompasses our mechanisms for taking in and interpreting our environment at the level of fact and feeling. It includes our thinking processes, our capacity to experience feelings, and our sense of self-worth.

Mental health refers to the health-fullness of your thinking—the limberness of your mind, your logic patterns, your problem-solving skills, your sense of humor, your creativity, your curiosity, your process for labeling and organizing your life experience.

In meeting and balancing the daily demands of life, mentally healthy people cope with problems as they arise, accept responsibility, welcome new experiences and new ideas, use their natural capacities, think for themselves and make their own decisions, put forth their best efforts, and find all these activities satisfying.

Emotional well-being is a second component of mental

health—your capacity to feel deeply, your sensitivity to feelings, your willingness to experience feelings, your motivations, the appropriateness of your responses, and your intuition. Mentally balanced people can usually cope with emotions—fear, anger, love, jealousy, guilt, or worry—and take life's disappointments in stride.

Self-respect is the third ingredient for mental well-being—your level of self-awareness, your attitude toward your strengths and limitations, your internal standards. Mentally healthy people know themselves and feel comfortable with themselves and others. They exhibit a confidence and trust in their capacity to deal with whatever situation comes along.

Does all this sound a bit heavy? Who could be all of this all of the time? No one! No one has all the characteristics of good mental health all of the time. Everyone experiences disappointments and fears, anxiety and doubt, ups and downs. Mental health does not mean perfection. Instead, it reflects the decision to live life openly and fully, acknowledging your limitations and affirming your strengths.

What about you? How would you rank your overall mental health?

Mental Health Inventory

- Do you feel in control of yourself?_____
- Can you laugh easily? Do you laugh each day?_____
- Can you cry easily? When was the last time? _____
- Give yourself a grade for common sense.   A   B   C   D   F
- Comment on your mental health level today. _____

  _____

Mental health requires the capacity to think clearly, the willingness to experience your feelings fully, and the esteem to trust yourself. The rest of the chapter looks at each of these dimensions more closely and pinpoints some strategies for self-care.

Explore your intellect

Daily life requires us to process and retain enormous quantities of information. Fortunately, the brain is a storage and retrieval system many times more complicated and efficient than the most complex computer. Remembering phone numbers, keeping appointments in mind, planning menus, listening to your children—these tasks may be routine but they all require substantial mental alertness. Figuring your income tax, tailoring a suit, driving a car, and giving a speech demand a bit more concentration. Our minds allow us to absorb, sort, and process hundreds of thousands of bits of data each day—data which we then combine in the correct way to tie our shoes or read a street sign or unlock our bicycle.

Although we may not be able to create an Adam out of dust, our intellect supplies us with the power to be creative. When we mix and synthesize and combine bits and pieces of our world, recasting them into some form that's new—at least for us—we're creating. We come up with a novel idea or give old ideas a new twist. We intuit the connections between events or people. We solve problems. We daydream. We see the incongruity around us and laugh. Our intellect allows us to be creative and to maintain a balanced outlook on life.

Consider for a moment your current mental functioning—your ability to think. Circle the appropriate number for each question on the Thinking Assessment.

Thinking Assessment

	very low				very high
How creative are you in seeing new options?	1	2	3	4	5
How good is your memory?	1	2	3	4	5
How curious are you?	1	2	3	4	5
How active is your imagination and fantasy?	1	2	3	4	5
How well do you concentrate?	1	2	3	4	5
How humorous or clever are you?	1	2	3	4	5
How well do you make judgments?	1	2	3	4	5

The answers to these questions are qualitative, not quantitative. They're relative to your personal capacities and limitations. An IQ of 130 doesn't insure mental health. Nor does one of 80 preclude creativity. There is no absolute standard or final destination.

Learning is a lifelong process of absorbing and forgetting, relearning and remembering, focusing and drifting, connecting, disconnecting and reconnecting. The assumption that we peak mentally at age 18 is absurd!

If you're interested in maintaining a vigorous intellectual fitness plan, consider including the following strategies into your self-care routine.

Four steps to a lively mind

Keep your thinking cap on. A public-service announcement reminds us, "a mind is a terrible thing to waste." Our minds need to be nourished just like our bodies. Read books. Ask questions. Explore. Experiment and grasp every opportunity to "fill'er up!"

Accept and meet new challenges willingly. Every problem is a challenge turned inside out. Every change can become stimulating as you seek to find ways to adjust. Be curious. Seek out new information. Challenge yourself to make tough decisions from which you will learn. Changing jobs, accepting new responsibilities, writing an article or speech, or taking a course can be an adventure—if you make it one.

Control your energy output. When you're overburdened, it's important to start limiting your investments. Choose to say "no" to some possibilities. Say it before you're empty, while you still have some reserve in your tank. Save some of your energy for yourself. When you're bored or underburdened, say "yes!" Seek out a new commitment, cause, or friendship.

Cultivate creativity. Stretch your imagination. Take a new route to church. Make up a story. State your problem in 10 different ways. Ask open-ended questions. Try a new recipe, or an old recipe with a new ingredient. Look for alternatives. Exaggerate your dilemma. Rearrange your office or your junk drawer or your priorities. Watch for the incongruities—and laugh! You can double your energy when you add a creative twist.

Investigate your emotions

Mental health is characterized by a wide variety of clear, strong feelings: irritation, anger, rage, excitement, anxiety, worry; despair, disappointment, sadness; joy, affection, arousal, love. To the extent that we allow ourselves to experience fully our whole range of feelings, we move toward the healthy balance.

It is tempting to manipulate our experiences to meet our desires or expectations, screening out "bad" feelings and acknowledging only "good" ones, or vice versa—tempting, but dangerous. While extreme ups and downs may be disruptive to life, or may even signal underlying problems that need to be resolved, the pursuit of emotional stability at any cost is probably even less healthy. People who are always moderate, never ruffled, and always even-keeled are probably shutting out or at least toning down some feelings. Unfortunately, feelings are rather rebellious creatures, and when we deny them they often go underground only to burst out at some later, usually inappropriate, time and place.

This does not mean that temper tantrums or promiscuity are mentally healthy. Angry feelings can be experienced without being expressed directly or destructively. Sexual attraction can be enjoyed without being indulged. Emotional health does require awareness of feelings. Paying attention to the signals our psyche sends us allows us to experience the depth and breadth of our emotional capacity.

We need not be at the mercy of our bodily sensations and psychic impulses. Feelings are controlled by our mind, not by external events. We create our feelings and reactions based on the way we interpret what's going on around us.

If we view a situation as a threat, feelings of hurt, fear, anger, and pain will follow. If we view it as a treat, feelings of comfort, joy, belonging, and anticipation will result. If we really want to

SEEKING YOUR HEALTHY BALANCE

feel differently, all we need is a new set of glasses for viewing the world.

A note of caution. An outburst of negative feelings may simply be your warning system signaling that something in your life is not right.

If you experience sudden, sharp abdominal pain, you probably will want to check out the source of the problem.

The same applies to emotional pain. Rather than denying the feelings, pay attention to their implicit request that you take a look at your life and see what's gone haywire. Check with a mental health professional who can help you understand the meaning in your emotional symptoms, and who can suggest strategies for helping you regain your emotional balance.

How about you? How healthily do you deal with your emotions?

Emotional Assessment

- How wide is your emotional spectrum?_____

- What feelings do you tend to screen out?_____

  _____

  _____

- Which feelings are your most frequent companions? _____

  _____

  _____

Three tips for feeling "good"

As you seek a healthy balance in your emotional well-being, you may want to try these ideas that have been suggested by mental health experts.

Stretch your feeling capacity. Feelings are at the heart of life. Yet most of us lack the vocabulary to distinguish and describe the subtle nuances of our experiences. Shades of love include affection, tenderness, admiration, liking, attraction, caring. We may hate, despise, dislike, or feel indifferent. Attraction may take the form of desire, longing, craving, coveting, or hankering. Hope leads us to anticipate, trust, rely, feel confident. Despair may take the form of desperation, despondency, doubt, suspicion, discouragement, disappointment, defeat, helplessness.

Next time you feel frightened, try to pinpoint the exact color and intensity of your emotion. Are you paralyzed? Anxious? Apprehensive? Panicky? Scared stiff? Terrified? Aroused? Exhilarated? Worried? Troubled? Disquieted? Uneasy? Appalled? Timid? Alarmed? Petrified? Jumpy? As you expand your feeling-word vocabulary, you may be surprised to discover a new depth and richness in your experiences.

Look for the silver linings. Choose to be positive. Every coin has two sides; every experience both a cost and a benefit; every life, an up side and a down side. Choose a positive mental attitude. Trust in yourself. Trust in your life. Saying, "everything will work out OK in the end," is phony only if you do nothing to help it work out. Laugh rather than complain. Play "ain't it funny" rather than "ain't it awful." Pop mental bubbles with humor.

Practice the attitude of gratitude. To a great extent our attitude determines the kinds of feelings we experience. A cynical, fearful, negative attitude will fill us with negative experience. A positive, hopeful, open attitude will fill us with warmth.

Hans Selye, the pioneer of stress research, claimed that hate and revenge are harmful to our physical health, while optimal physical functioning is associated with the attitude of gratitude. Poisoning your life by attempting to get even hurts only you. "I'll get you, if it's the last thing I do" may very well be the last thing you do! Obsession with hate and revenge erodes our bodies, our minds, and our spirits—not to mention our relationships with others. Love and thankfulness will open your life and fill it with vitality and healing.

Develop your sense of self

One of the best ways to stay mentally healthy is to know, respect, and like yourself. In short, to maintain a healthy self-concept.

For some of us that's no easy task. We bombard ourselves with a nonstop commentary on our thoughts, feelings, behavior, appearance: "You klutz!" "Simmer down now," "Next to her you look like a tank," "Stupid!" "You never finish anything," "You'd better not!" "She doesn't like me," "He thinks I'm empty-headed," "That's crazy," "If you were a stronger person you could stop," "You creep," "You're never going to make it." It's tough to keep a sense of perspective in the face of all those critical messages.

Fortunately, this irrational self-talk is often contradicted by feedback from others and from the environment—and occasionally even from within ourselves. Our worst fears are not confirmed. You move gracefully through the room. He praises your memo. She invites you to play racquetball. Your "crazy" idea inspires a new ad campaign. You do make it. Somehow we survive these mental gymnastics, some of us with more self-esteem than others.

We all have our own levels of intelligence, our own strengths and limitations, our own emotional patterns and personal characteristics that contribute to our own sense of self. When we can authentically affirm all these dimensions of self, including our inadequacies, we are better able to meet life's challenges. With a positive self-concept we can face up to the problems we encounter, feeling confident and optimistic about our capacity to cope effectively with them.

How about you? How healthy is your self-esteem?

Self-Esteem Assessment

- In what ways does your positive view of yourself enhance your well-being? _____

_____

_____

- What are some of your favorite personal putdowns? _____

_____

_____

- What qualities of yours do you particularly admire? _____

_____

_____

Most of us need a periodic boost for recharging our self-confidence. The strategies for promoting self-esteem outlined below can help you take better care of yourself!

Six self-esteem builders

Talk to yourself gently. Are you your own worst critic? What do you say to yourself as you go through your day? Call yourself bad names and you'll end up a lot more fatigued than if you whisper sweet somethings. Remember the last time you were embarrassed. Did you say to yourself, "Oh, you dummy, look what a fool you are!"? Why not change that self-talk to, "Look at all the attention I'm getting," or, "It's OK, I learn from my mistakes." Instead of saying, "I want everyone to like me," why not say, "Ninety-nine percent is good enough." Instead of, "I should get everything I want when I want it!" why not say, "I'll never get all that I want." Do you get the point? Try to counter your irrational self-talk with positive messages that let you off the hook.

Be realistic. Accept your limits as part of your humanness, not as blemishes to be eradicated. So you have a high-pitched voice. So your mind is boggled by numbers. So your foot turns out. So your hair is coarse. So you don't like everyone you meet. So you can't act on all your ideas. So what! If no one else notices your good points, pat yourself on the back. Sprinkle your shortcomings with a grain of salt. Avoid comparisons—especially with an "ideal you" based on everyone else's best traits.

Worry wisely. Avoid worrying prematurely about what might happen in the future. When Angie and John anxiously pressed their doctor about how long their diabetic son might live, he wisely replied, "If you cross the bridge before you get there, you'll have to pay the toll twice." When you can't control the outcome, let go. Mark Twain once said, "I've seen a great many problems in life and most of them never happened."

Surrender! Some things you simply can't change. You aren't God. Don't hit your head against a stone wall. When you can influence the outcome, worry only long enough to warm up for action. Try to live without regrets. Surrender to the flow of life. Let go and laugh.

Affirm your resources. Attend to your internal sources of strength. Keep them in mind and make them work for you, whatever they are. Mother Teresa, a model of caring in the 20th century, was once asked, "What are the sources of your strength?" She replied, "A 98-year-old woman in Philadelphia who prays for me." Strength is around you and within you. If you get centered and bring your strength alive in your mind, it will work for you. Spend some time alone with yourself, centering in on your internal resources.

Focus on what deeply satisfies you. Occupy yourself and your time with projects, commitments, challenges, and people that help you feel worthwhile. Don't just put in time laboring at repetitious or meaningless work. Even if you have to "labor" to keep a roof over your head, spend as much energy as possible in your "lifework." Invest yourself in some creative, meaningful activity that gives you a sense of purpose and worth. You may volunteer respite care for parents of a handicapped child or telephone for United Way or work your 40 hours in critical care. For mental health it's important that you're able to say, "I'm useful," "I held up my end," "I did good!"

Hang in there when the going gets tough. When you feel as if your world is falling apart and you think you're going to pieces, don't withdraw from your meaningful commitments. If you do, you'll feel useless and you'll just confirm your sense of falling to pieces. Try to keep performing your responsibilities as normally as possible. Tell yourself, "I'm strong enough," "I can manage," "I will grow from this experience."

Before moving on to consider relational self-care, please stop and reflect on your overall mental self-care habits. Do they enhance or erode your well-being?

Personal Reflection on My Mental Health

■ My intellectual patterns (curiosity, learning, creativity, openness to challenges, control of energy investment) _____

_____

■ My emotional patterns (acceptance and range of feelings, positive outlook, gratitude, revenge)

_____

■ My self-esteem patterns (internal dialogs, worry, strengths, meaningful work, affirmations)

_____

_____

Wish List for My Mental Health

■ List here everything you can imagine wanting for your mental health. What would you like to be able to do? To know? To feel? To learn? Let your imagination run free. Don't limit yourself in any way. The wishes don't have to be practical. Have fun dreaming.

I wish I could: _____

_____

_____

_____

_____

5

FILL ME with LOVE

Relational self-care

In the early 60s Sidney Jourard hypothesized that people who loved deeply would live longer. This pioneer in the field of intentional relationship-building believed that if we revealed ourselves to one another we would live vital, high-energy lives with less sickness and suffering.

Jourard's theory has recently been substantiated by the results of a longitudinal study of "healthy" men. These 200 men were followed for 40 years after graduation from college to determine what factors would distinguish the healthy group from those who were disabled or deceased. Surprisingly, the crucial difference was not salt intake or exercise or weight control. The key to health was self-disclosure. The healthy group reported the consistent presence in their lives of at least one individual with whom they could share their thoughts and feelings. For some men this sympathetic ear belonged to a spouse; for others it was a friend or colleague.

Isolation is sickening

This study reinforces what common sense and folk wisdom has known for centuries: loneliness and alienation make people sick. In Old Testament times a person excluded from community was considered to be dead. Today, in a similar way people still sicken and die outside of human community.

Choosing to develop rich and meaningful relationships is a vital survival skill. A supportive network of friends who offer understanding, closeness, and fellowship enhances your potential for well-being.

How about you? Use the worksheet on the next page to help you review your support network.

Relationship Inventory

- How many people know you deeply and understand who you really are? Name at least one—five or six would be better. _____, _____,

  _____, _____, _____,

  _____, _____, _____

- Look at your list of supporters and reflect on the different ways you have of letting each of these people know you. _____

  _____

  _____

Develop healthy relationships

Healthy relationships are characterized by reciprocal responsibilities and mutual satisfaction. When two people are committed to give and take, to sharing and listening, the needs of both are satisfied in the exchange. This chapter focuses on self-care, looking at the receiving side of relationships. The giving dimension is covered in later chapters on reaching out.

If you find it difficult to focus on your own needs rather than on those of others, remember the results of the study. The healthy men actively sought out relationships that would meet their needs. So can you. And you can reap the same reward—health.

Reflect for a moment on the current health of your relationships with others, then respond to the questions below.

Relationship Assessment

- How fulfilling were your interactions with others this past week?

	Frequently	Occasionally	Never
Did you feel alone even when you were with others?	_____	_____	_____
Did you feel rejected? Ignored? Let down?	_____	_____	_____
Did you feel that people misunderstood or didn't appreciate you?	_____	_____	_____
Did you feel isolated? Without support?	_____	_____	_____
Did you feel forgotten? Left out? Uninvolved?	_____	_____	_____
Did you feel pressured? Overburdened with responsibility to others?	_____	_____	_____
Did you feel drained? As if you'd given your last ounce of caring?	_____	_____	_____

- Summarize how you feel about your relationships during this past week, and how successfully they nurtured you. _____

_____

_____

Everyone feels unsupported once in a while. However, if these feelings are familiar and frequent for you, it may be a sign that you need to work on improving your support network. The self-care suggestions on the following pages may help you nurture the health of your relationships.

Practice self-disclosure

Sharing yourself with others is a matter of choice, not chance. Some people choose openness; others tend to hide their inner selves. Each of us faces the decision hundreds of times each day: "Shall I say what's really in my heart and share myself as I really am inside, or not?" "Should I maintain my public self, or let my private self sneak out?"

People who keep up a good front, never talking about their problems and deepest fears, cut themselves off from a major source of healing and support. What you won't share with anyone else is usually something you need to hear, something you are unwilling to accept about you. When you succeed in putting up a good front, you lose touch with yourself and your heart.

Excuses for not sharing are endless: "He won't be interested," "They won't understand," "Don't wash your dirty linen in public," "I'm not that close to anyone," "My life is just too hectic, there's no time," "She's got more troubles than I have." All are potentially accurate statements, but not good excuses for closing yourself off.

Obviously, it's inappropriate to "spill your guts" indiscriminately. Sometimes it's better to keep your mouth shut. But most of the time with some special people, or some of the time with most people, you need to share yourself—for your benefit. It's just too exhausting to maintain your public self all the time. We all need someone—at least one someone—who knows and accepts our private self, too.

How about you? Stop and reflect on how adequately you are sharing your deepest feelings.

Self-Disclosure Assessment

- In what ways is your public self different from your private self? _____
  _____

- How much of yourself are you willing to share with:

  Your spouse?_____ Your children?_____
  Your parents?_____ Your best friend?_____
  Your work associates?_____ People in general?_____

- What would you be unwilling to share with these particular people? _____
  _____
  _____

- What kinds of things have you never shared with anyone? (Use a secret code if you wish.)

  Your inner most fears? _____

  A painful experience? _____

  Something of which you aren't proud?_____

  Your greatest joys or accomplishments? _____

- Pick one of these private aspects of yourself and determine to disclose that experience to someone during the next week.

  What will you share?_____

  Whom will you tell it to?_____

  When will you do it? _____

A note of warning: if you know that what you want to share would be hurtful to the other person, find someone else to listen to this particular feeling or experience. It's tempting to use sharing as retaliation. That's not appropriate.

Know your needs

Each of us has a variety of interpersonal needs. To feel connected with others we must be plugged into a support network that satisfies these needs. Interpersonal support may come from many sources and take many forms, but all of us require that our basic needs be met on a regular basis.

Sometimes we just need the support of someone who will listen intently to whatever is on our mind or in our heart. Paul Tournier, Swiss theologian and physician, reflected, "It is impossible to overemphasize the immense need people have to be really listened to, to be taken seriously, to be understood."

At other times we need emotional nurture, the unconditional positive regard that lets us know beyond any doubt that we are loved and cherished—just as we are, without one plea.

Support may also take the form of feedback, honest information that gives us an opportunity to check our perception of reality with someone else. This kind of mirror-holding is a rare gift when we ask for it and when we respect the giver. It's a little less easy to take when it's unsolicited.

Whether our lifework is parenting or painting or providing services to others, each of us needs interpersonal support to sustain and enrich our on-the-job efforts. On occasion we need commendation, positive feedback about our skills and accomplishments. We need to be praised for a job well done and appreciated for our unique contributions.

As in the personal arena, we all need challenge, feedback, and information that stimulates us to stretch and grow. Although it's tough to listen to criticism without defensiveness, to learn about ourselves, we all need to be challenged.

Finally, all of us need someone with whom we can share laughter and play time, satisfying our need for re-creation.

Who fills these interpersonal needs for you? One person? Several people? Different people at different times? Think of all the people you know and interact with: friends, work associates, close family, relatives, church acquaintances, neighbors, clients, store clerks, service people, club members. All of these relationships serve a purpose, meet some need for you. They can potentially be a source of interpersonal support and vitalization, or a source of disappointment.

Complete the following Interpersonal Needs Assessment to evaluate the health of your current support network.

Interpersonal Needs Assessment

■ How well are your interpersonal needs being met right now?

	To whom do you look?	How successfully are your needs met?	Who else could possibly fill this need?
Listening			
Emotional nurture			
Feedback			
Commendation			
Challenge			
Play			

■ What do you observe about your responses?

Do you rely on only one person? Are some of your important needs currently not being met? What might you like to strengthen or change? Note some of your observations.

_____

_____

_____

As you review your relationships from the need-fulfillment perspective, you may want to keep the following principles in mind.

Five principles for getting your needs met

Don't put all your eggs in one basket. It is extremely unlikely that one person can meet all your interpersonal needs. Don't depend on a single soul to function as your entire support network.

Don't beat your head against a stone wall. Frustration results when we expect an inappropriate person to meet a particular need. Don't bother looking for understanding and acceptance from someone you know can't or won't come through. Don't expect your workaholic roommate to take time out for jumping in a leaf pile.

Accept willing substitutes. Even if there's a vacant position (spouse, best friend, father confessor) in your life for a time, you can still find people to meet each of your interpersonal needs.

Don't wait for a mind reader. Intentionality is essential in human relationships. Know what you need and search out someone to help you satisfy that need. You have to reveal yourself to get your needs met. Ask for what you want. It's foolish to say to yourself, "If they really loved me they would know what I want without my asking." It's foolish to make other people guess what you need. When you do, you're less likely to receive what would fill you.

Speak up. It's risky to ask for what you want. Others might not give it to you. Or if they do, you may discover that it's not as satisfying as you had imagined. However, the risks of rejection and dissatisfaction seem small in comparison to the risks of isolation, loneliness, and frustration.

When you find yourself feeling isolated and lonely, it's likely that you're not getting all of what you need from others. It might be necessary for you to carefully analyze the support you're missing and intentionally fill the gaps in your relationships.

Know and nurture your support network

The average person meets well over 10,000 people in a lifetime—family, colleagues at work, church members, neighbors, sales clerks, teachers, fellow students, public figures, auto mechanics, friends, friends of friends. Our contacts increase in ever-wider ripples, expanding our potential support network.

Most people don't intentionally convert that potential into an actuality. Unless you clearly identify your support network, you probably won't take steps to nurture it and help it grow. You are surrounded by hundreds of pairs of smiling eyes waiting to be drafted into your army of supporters. Who are they?

Identify your network of family and friends by completing the following exercise.

Circles of Support

- Draw a chart of your support network by using this circle.

  Put your name in the inner circle.

  Think first about the persons with whom you have the strongest bonds. Write their names in the circle around you.

  In the outer circle add people with whom you have less frequent or more casual contact.

  Continue diagramming and adding names as long as you can. Then use your address book or photograph album to jog your memory some more. List as many people as you like.

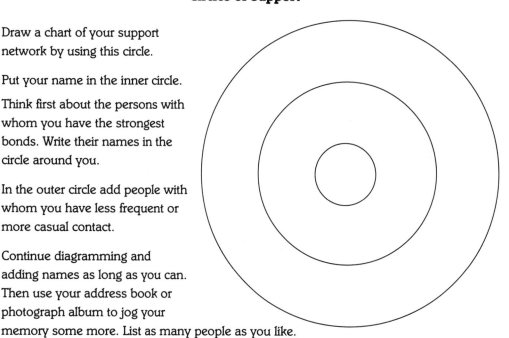

  Think about each person in the diagram and remember the closeness you've shared.

  Pick one or two people you'd especially like to have positive contact with right now. Plan to make that contact via phone or in person during the next 24 hours.

- Who have you selected for positive contact? _____

- How will you plan to make that contact happen within the next 24 hours?

  _____

  _____

  _____

Start a support group

One effective strategy for assuring that you'll get the personal support you need is to start a group.

A support group is a gathering of people who make a commitment to meet regularly and to listen, share, and care. A bowling team may be supportive, but it's not a support group. A coffee circle may be supportive, but it's not a support group either. A support group is an intentional gathering for the direct purpose of relating to and learning from each other.

A group like this involves equal exchange among peers. There is no designated leader and no status hierarchy. When choosing support group members, pick people you think would be helpful to you. They don't have to be your best friends. Some people you hardly know could be excellent sources of feedback and learning for you. Remember, this group is for you. Don't select people who you think would benefit from a group unless they also can meet some of your needs.

The basis of the group—the glue, if you will—is commitment over time. Plan to meet together at least twice a month for six months. Make the support group a top priority.

Here are some tips for how to make sure that your group is, in fact, really supportive.

Be ready to share yourself. In sharing yourself you learn to know yourself more fully.

Be ready to support and be supported. Support starts with your presence and careful listening.

Give yourselves time to become a group. Don't hurry. Take time to tell your stories, to get acquainted in depth.

Make a clear contract. Agree on how you will listen to each

other, share feelings, solve problems, respect off-limit areas, and maintain confidentiality.

Give no feedback unless it's asked for. A support group is not an encounter group, and it's not therapy, although it may be therapeutic. Unsolicited feedback is not appropriate. Keep it to yourself.

Know that the needs of the people in the group will change. Set periodic times to reevaluate individual needs and redefine your contract with one another.

Potential Support Group Recruits

■ If you were to start a support group, whom would you like to invite?

_____, _____, _____

_____, _____, _____

_____, _____, _____

_____, _____, _____

Don't be afraid to risk. Some people you ask will be interested and others won't. Gather those who are interested. Make your commitment to one another, and see what happens over the months. You might like to begin by sharing about your healthy balance dilemmas, using the Thought Provokers at the end of this book.

Watch out for people traps

Although relationships can be wonderful health enhancers, it's also easy to get caught in unhealthy relationship patterns that sap your energy and leave you unfulfilled and fatigued. Beware of these three typical tangles.

Pleasing others. If you try to please everyone and make sure everyone always approves of you 100 percent, you're 100 percent guaranteed to end up exhausted and disappointed. Trying to please everyone is an impossible goal, a no-win endeavor!

Taking on too much responsibility. If you seldom say "no," requests from others may soon overwhelm you. This is just another form of trying to please everyone. To stay healthy you'll have to learn to limit yourself to caring only for those most important to you.

This trap catches many of us in the middle years when we're surrounded by demands from growing children and from aging parents, both generations struggling with dependence and independence. When you're in that spot, it's understandable that you sometimes feel exhausted and discouraged. Try not to add anyone else to your caring list at that point. Your hands are already full. In a few more years you'll be ready to volunteer for relationship duty again. For the present time, find some ways to get your own needs met.

Playing the game of "Poor Lonely Me." Loneliness comes from being alone when you don't want to be. It hurts, but it's not the end of the world, and it doesn't have to be permanent.

Withdrawing into your shell and feeling sorry for yourself will only perpetuate the problem and won't get you much sympathy anyway. So, take action on your own behalf.

First, accept the fact that you're lonely, and let the feelings be. Don't try to change them with eating, drinking, surface relationships, or irresponsible sex. Just accept yourself as you are right now.

Second, find someone you can talk to about your feelings. Confide in someone—even if you have to pay a therapist to listen.

Third, experiment with changes in your patterns of living that will help break down your isolation. If you haven't found a way to meet another best friend, then try volunteering with the elderly or reading books to the blind. Don't sit at home waiting for someone to come to you. Reach out in some way to break out of your loneliness.

Do any of these people traps sound familiar? Are any of them currently disturbing your healthy balance?

Relationship Traps Assessment

■ Have you fallen into any of the three costly people traps?

Pleasing others? _____ When?_____

Taking on too much responsibility? _____ When? _____

Playing the game of "Poor Lonely Me"? _____ When? _____

■ What negative effects have these traps caused in your relationships with others?

_____

_____

■ What might you wish to try differently? _____

_____

_____

_____

Before moving on to consider spiritual self-care, please stop
and think through your patterns of relating to others. Do your
current relationships and your relationship habits enhance or
erode your level of well-being?

Personal Reflection on My Relationship Health

■ My self-disclosure patterns: _____

■ My basic need fulfillment:_____

■ My support network:_____

■ My negative habits (traps): _____

Wish List for My Relationship Health

■ List here everything you can imagine wanting for your relational health. What would you feel
like? Who would you relate to? Who would you like to meet? Let your imagination run free.
Don't limit yourself in any way. The wishes don't have to be practical. Have fun dreaming.

I wish I could: _____

_____

_____

_____

_____

6

MAGIC MOMENTS
Spiritual self-care

Back in the 50s, the Hollywood fad was 3-D movies. With your ticket you received a pair of cardboard glasses with one green lens and one red. These remarkable contraptions brought a third dimension to movie viewing—depth.

Spiritual reality is the depth dimension of life. In order to focus on this aspect of whole person well-being, you'll need your own set of 3-D glasses, with its matching vocabulary. Your spectacles give you a particular viewpoint and words for bringing your spiritual beliefs into focus. You learn to describe your experience and endow it with meaning in a way that seems comfortable and proper to you. Your perspective and language, whatever they are, are your spiritual tools.

No particular set of glasses is the correct one for all. So get out your own belief spectacles, and polish them up so that you can view your spiritual health at its maximum depth, color, and impact. Feel free to translate the examples in this book as necessary into whatever language and images are meaning-full to you.

The spirit connection

Health and wholeness are essentially spiritual concepts. In general, Americans haven't spent much time focusing on the spiritual dimension of life. Consequently, we don't know as much about health and wholeness as we'd like. The time has come for us to accept the spiritual as an important—perhaps the most important—dimension of well-being.

Most of us know intuitively that medical treatments, or any of the self-care remedies we've examined so far, are not powerful enough to heal us if our spirit is fractured. We all know people whose physical health has failed because they've lost purpose in life. We know others whose guilt feelings are so profound that mental health or satisfying relationships seem like unattainable goals.

The power of the spirit manifests itself even more dramatically in the many inspiring accounts of people whose faith has made them whole. A young mother miraculously survived a life-threatening illness and surgery. None of the physicians expected her to live. The anesthesiologist came to visit her three times before she left the hospital. Each time he said things like, "Some things you just can't explain," and, "You have an extraordinary will to live." It was obvious that his medical knowledge couldn't explain to him why she had not died. The activity of the spirit and the will, along with hope, can be catalysts that mobilize our healing resources in ways that our reason cannot understand.

The Swiss psychiatrist Carl Jung was convinced that spiritual concerns are the central components of health. He observed:

> Among my patients in the second half of life there has not been one whose problem in the last resort was not that of finding a religious outlook on life . . . and none of them really has been healed who did not regain his religious outlook.

Jesus' ministry was filled with incidents that clearly connected health with the human spirit. The blind were given their sight, the lame could walk again, the troubled were purged of "demons," social outcasts were welcomed into fellowship. All were healed on the strength of their belief and their contrite hearts—their spiritual health.

Your values, beliefs, and commitments can be the keys to your health as well. The spiritual dimension of life can be either a source of distress or a powerful resource for health.

What is spiritual health?

Although religious beliefs and practices may contribute to spiritual health, spiritual health is by no means determined only by the rituals and dogma of the organized church. The word spiritual is used here to refer to that core dimension of you—your innermost self—that provides you with a profound sense of who you are, where you came from, where you're going, and how you might reach your goal.

In addition to supplying meaning for life, the spiritual dimension provides you with principles for living and explains to you why the universe works the way it does. Commitment to God or some ultimate concern engenders a spirit of selflessness, sensitivity to others, and a willingness to sacrifice for people in need.

The spiritual dimension of life recognizes a power beyond the natural and rational, accepts on faith the unknown or difficult to explain, and provides a framework for understanding death. Rituals and ceremonies create structures for attending to and expressing our spiritual selves. Our spirituality is the key to helping us make the tough healthy balance decisions.

How about you? Use the following assessment to reflect on your current level of spiritual well-being.

Spiritual Well-Being Assessment

- To what extent are you attuned to your spiritual core? Do you consider yourself:

  A deep person? _____

  A spirit-filled person? _____

  A religious person? _____

  How? In what ways? _____

  _____

- What part does God play in your life? _____

- Would you say you are spiritually healthy? _____

- Compare the qualities of spiritual health and spiritual atrophy listed below. Circle the words in each pair that best describe your current spiritual condition or add words that fit you better. Which collection more accurately describes your current condition?

Spiritual Health	Spiritual Atrophy
hope	emptiness
positive outlook	anxiety
acceptance of death	loss of meaning
forgiveness, self acceptance	self-judgment, self-condemnation
commitment	apathy
meaning and purpose	long "dry" spells
clear values	conflicting values
sense of worth	needing to prove myself
peace	harried and hurried
in touch with God	dead at the core
worship, prayer, meditation	without rituals that touch me

- Observations—comments to yourself _____

  _____

  _____

  _____

No matter what your present position on the atrophy/health continuum, there are positive steps you can take to enhance your spiritual health and consequently your overall well-being.

Get in touch with your core

Who are you? Where did you come from? Where are you going? When all the surface layers are peeled away, what do you believe is at the core of life? What is at the core of you?

The process of touching and being touched by your core is an experience that creates wholeness and gives you energy. When people are out of touch with what's central in life—focusing on the periphery—they become dis-spirited and de-energized.

Enthusiasm, that bubbling of life energy, comes from tapping into the spirit of God within—deep within. The Greek root word for enthusiasm means "in God"—in touch with the energy of the divine, filled with and able to express God's energy as it flows through. When you're in touch with that energy, you know you're alive. Today we use enthusiasm to mean fervent, passionate, positive mental interest, and we have almost forgotten the divine spirit meaning—but it's still there.

At times people are receptive to spiritual reflection, at other times they are not. At times spiritual realities barge in on our lives and we are ready to deal with them. At other times we are not ready and don't sense the need at all.

How do you go about getting in touch with your core? For starters, you can set up an atmosphere that helps you get ready and that invites spiritual reflection.

The five postures for spiritual growth below suggest some strategies for tuning in to your spiritual core.

Five postures for spiritual growth

Be quiet. Spiritual truths often come in the form of a still small voice that is difficult to hear above the chaos and confusion of a frantic lifestyle. Set aside time for solitude and meditation.

Be open to the spiritual. Spiritual experiences often come in unexpected forms and packages. They surprise us. Foster a non-judgmental attitude so that you're open to the spiritual dimension in any life event—from hoeing the garden to witnessing an accident, from watching a swim meet to reading the morning paper. God may be waiting in the wings to touch your core.

Be inquisitive and curious. An attitude of active searching increases your options and your potential for spiritual centering. Don't shut doors before you check out what's behind them. For example, the laying on of hands may be a powerful centering experience. Through interpersonal Bible study you may discover whole new dimensions of yourself. A silent retreat might renew your enthusiasm. The study of meditation or the practice of yoga may very well allow you to experience tranquility and peace.

Be receptive to pain and grief. Pain helps us focus on the widest questions of our being. It's a deepener. A life without pain leads to a sparse, shallow existence. Allow yourself to feel your pain fully, then ask, "What is it trying to teach me?"

Be playful. Play is a pleasurable, freeing experience. It breeds spontaneous enthusiasm and celebration. When you make music, dance, laugh, sing—however you play—listen for sounds of the spirit.

Try seeing with your soul

Spiritual experiences take many forms. Can you recall moments when you felt centered, in touch with your deepest core? Times when you were touched by an eternal truth, knew you were on holy ground? At an evening worship experience? A moment of great sorrow at a death? A sunset? A storm? A word of forgiveness and love? A period of intense pain? A sense of unity with everything living?

Sometimes these touching moments are high "mountaintop" experiences; sometimes they are deep reflective experiences. But whether we sink deep into ourselves or soar out beyond our usual boundaries of the self, at these moments we are in touch with the eternal and have tapped into a source of energy much greater than ourselves.

Most spiritual experiences transcend the images of physical time and space that we typically call reality. At these moments we see beyond the limits. We see with our soul, not with our eyes. We know, not with the mind, but with the heart. This special knowledge and insight is a rare gift. Periodically we need to give ourselves space and quiet—to sit down by the side of the road and let our souls catch up to us.

Rediscover the depth dimension

Oil is discovered not by drilling a thousand one-foot holes, but by drilling one thousand-foot hole. We grow in spiritual vision by contemplating the meaning of the deepest, most touching moments of our lives—and by letting these experiences guide our vision and our decisions.

Recall a few of the most touching moments in your life.

Personal Depth Experiences

■ List some of your most touching, deep moments. What truth did you discover in each of these soul times:

Event_____ Truth _____

Event_____ Truth _____

Event_____ Truth _____

Event_____ Truth _____

Event_____ Truth _____

■ How did these experiences energize you? _____

_____

■ Describe the wisdom and perspective you gained in these special times of depth.

_____

■ How does this new view educate and guide your current decision making?_____

_____

_____

How can you stay in touch with these eternal truths and regularly promote your spiritual health? Most religious traditions suggest that the process of being in relationship with the Creator has health-giving potential. When we set aside time for reflection, meditation, and prayer, we provide opportunity for staying in touch with and being touched by the source of life and health.

What about you? Do you give yourself the reflection time that allows you to grow spiritually?

Quiet Time Assessment

- Do you provide space in your day for spiritual reflection? _____
- How satisfied are you with the level and quality of that commitment? _____
- In what ways could you act intentionally to increase your spiritual depth? _____

_____

_____

_____

Expand your images of health

As you expand your awareness of the spiritual dimension of health, you will discover more and more qualities that contribute to your wholeness and well-being. A dozen virtues that could potentially fill your life and enhance your health are listed on the next two pages. As you read them, consider each image carefully. Meditate on them one by one. Get a sense of the positive clarity and energy they provide for you as you make them the focus of your attention and allow them to fill you.

Twelve Elements of Spiritual Health

■ Comment on each of these spiritual qualities.

Love: the commitment to invest in another rather than remain self-engrossed.

To whom have you committed yourself in love? _____

_____

Intimacy: the choice to abandon isolation and independence in favor of heartfelt sharing, mutual support, and interdependence.

With whom are you intimate? _____

_____

Trust: the willingness to be vulnerable instead of cautious, suspicious, and cynical.

In what ways do you allow yourself to be vulnerable?_____

With whom?_____

Meaning: a clear sense of direction, no longer drifting without purpose.

What gives you a sense of direction? _____

Where are you headed? _____

Hope: the vision of a desirable future, a present pregnant with promise, eager to be born.

What is your vision of your future? _____

_____

Faith: the unquestioning leap of faith, relinquishing fear to affirm the not-yet-proven.

What are your convictions? _____

_____

Commitment: the decision to invest rather than straddle the fence, to move toward a goal.

Where have you invested yourself with strength and perseverance? _____

_____

Patience: the ability to wait, allowing the future its chance to emerge, no longer pushing the river to make life happen.

How and when do you wait expectantly and patiently? _____

_____

Joy: the rush of delight that fills an empty shell.

When do you let yourself bubble with joy? _____

_____

Imagination: the new view, the creative spark that challenges habit and boredom.

What would be some new options for you?   I could _____

I could _____   I could _____

Courage: the willingness to face limitations and still risk rather than playing it safe.

When have you ventured in spite of your limits?_____

_____

Gratitude: the thankful appreciation that counteracts the myth of self-sufficiency.

For what are you truly thankful? _____

_____

- After considering this evidence of depth in your life, how would you assess your current spiritual health? _____

_____

- Summarize the themes you see in your responses.

I see that_____

and _____

- Share your analysis and insights with someone you trust .

(Who?)_____(When?)_____

As you pay attention to caring for your spirit watch out for three main causes of spiritual atrophy.

Three cautions

Cynicism erodes the spirit. Cynicism closes down the spirit as effectively as a lethal herbicide. Although our spiritual nature is deep, its flowers are often fragile. When you feel a spell of cynicism coming on, look for something to cherish or celebrate instead.

Religious piety may hinder spiritual development. Religion or church activities may actually get in the way of spiritual experiences if we let them obscure the underlying meaning. Be careful when dogma becomes more important than depth, the trivial more important than the core. Rigid, narrow, judgmental thinking can close off opportunities for your spirit to stretch and grow.

A spirit ignored, withers. It's tempting to ignore the spirit dimension of life since the consequences of spirit-lessness usually don't show up until crisis points. Spirits suffer from inattention and neglect without complaint. They rust silently from lack of use. Don't count on your core for help in crises, unless you've nourished and exercised it regularly.

Please stop and consider again your overall patterns of spiritual self-care. Do your spiritual habits enhance or erode your level of well-being?

Personal Reflection on My Spiritual Health

- What values, beliefs, and commitments do I most cherish? _____

  _____

  How do these central spiritual truths enhance my health? _____

  _____

- Which aspects of spirit are missing or weak in my life? _____

  _____

- What rituals do I find meaningful and helpful for promoting my spiritual depth? _____

  _____

  How could I increase their healing effects? _____
- How does my spiritual health shape my healthy balance decisions? _____

  _____

- What advice could I give younger persons that might help them develop a richer spiritual life?

  _____

Wish List for My Spiritual Health

- List here everything you can imagine wanting for your spiritual health. How would you like to feel? Act? What would you like to be? Let your imagination run free. Don't limit yourself in any way. The wishes don't have to be practical. Have fun dreaming.

  I wish I could: _____

  _____

  _____

  _____

  _____

7

PUTTING the PIECES TOGETHER

A wholistic view

Assess your self-care

How effective are your current self-care patterns? Do your habits help you maintain a balance that's healthy for you? One person answered these questions this way:

"Physically, I'm operating at about 70%. I have lots of energy, but with my sore knee I haven't been able to exercise as I'd like. I'm sleeping well and am relaxed."

"Mentally, I'm not very stimulated. I'm bored at work and waiting for a new challenge."

"My relationships are so-so. I'm depending on just one person to meet most of my interpersonal needs and I'm not getting much feedback or challenge from anyone."

"Spiritually, I'm in super shape! God is at the center of my life and guides my choices. Prayer is a daily solace and resource. I do wonder sometimes, though, if I'm too judgmental."

"Overall I'd say that, while I'm doing well, I probably should balance my self-care habits by getting more exercise and by finding new and stimulating challenges that will stretch my thinking."

As these responses indicate, the answers to the balance questions are complex, and they are unique for each of us.

What about you? How is your whole person well-being? Would you say you're currently maintaining a healthy balance? You may want to leaf through the first half of this book to jog your memory about insights you had while reading. If you took notes or wrote in a journal, scan those as well for your self-care assessment. Then answer the following questions to assess your current health status.

Your Current Health Status Assessment

- Comment on your current level of well-being in all aspects of life. Be very specific. Use examples whenever possible.

  Physical Health: I'm_____

  _____

  Mental Health: I'm_____

  _____

  Relational Health: I'm _____

  _____

  Spiritual Health: I'm_____

  _____

- Complete the sentence: I feel most alive when _____

  _____

- Aspects of my health I would like to improve:_____

  _____

- Complete the following statement: If I want my health to improve,

  I need to stop_____

  and I need to start _____

- Comment on your general satisfaction/dissatisfaction with your total health at this moment.

  _____

  _____

  _____

What are your health priorities?

What did you notice as you answered the Health Status questions? You may have discovered that the quality of your health and self-care habits differs among the four dimensions. Rarely do people invest equal amounts of energy in mental, spiritual, relational, and physical health.

Each of us determines which aspects are most important to us. We pay special attention to these. One person, for example, might not care much about the ability to think abstractly, but might place high value on physical fitness. Another loves good friends and desires spiritual depth, but doesn't give a hoot about physical conditioning or nutrition.

We all target some aspects of health for special attention, based on our values and priorities. What about you? Is mental health more important to you than spiritual depth? Is physical health more important than friendship? Use the questions below to discover your priorities.

Health Priority Ranking

- Rank each aspect of health in order of its importance to you. Assign #1 to the most important, #2 to the next most important, etc. This forced-choice ranking may be difficult, but it should also help you see what you value most in personal health.

    _____ Physical Health (strength, energy, freedom from pain, endurance)

    _____ Mental Health (memory, humor, good judgment, stability, calmness)

    _____ Relational Health (many friends, loving, caring, good contact)

    _____ Spiritual Health (peace, hope, confidence, purpose, faith)

- What aspect of health should you focus on improving right now? _____

Favorite symptoms

The health priorities you select determine which symptoms you'll pay attention to and which ones you'll ignore. Most of us have enough symptoms of ill health to call ourselves sick most of the time. We also have enough signs of wholeness to call ourselves healthy.

The symptom you first notice is not necessarily the first that occurs, just the first you're willing to attend to. Some people get worried about a queasy stomach or changes in their skin long before they even notice the diminished meaningful contact with friends. They're more likely to call a physician for a prescription than a neighbor for coffee and conversation. Other people are particularly attuned to their mood signals so that depression or anxiety is more troublesome to them than arthritis. They can ignore physical pain much more easily than psychic pain.

It's even possible to manipulate symptoms until you can pick the ones that you want. A father once said, "My daughter knows that if she's discouraged or worried, she still must go to school, but if she has a high temperature, she can stay home. She can raise her temperature any time she wants to. You know how I know? I used to do it to my mother."

How about you? If you have to be sick which symptoms do you prefer?

Favorite Symptoms Ranking

- Brainstorm "sickness" symptoms that you might typically experience in the four dimensions of well-being. List at least five in each area.

Body	Mind	Relationships	Spirit
headache	prejudice	arguments	arrogance
fever	depression	rebellion	hopelessness
_____	_____	_____	_____
_____	_____	_____	_____
_____	_____	_____	_____
_____	_____	_____	_____
_____	_____	_____	_____
_____	_____	_____	_____

- Go back and circle the symptoms you're most likely to experience.

  Are they primarily physical, mental, relational, or spiritual? _____

- Which symptoms are least acceptable to you? _____

  _____

- Which do you ignore? _____

  _____

- Which will cause you to take immediate corrective action? _____

  _____

- Observations/insights/reflections on what you have written_____

  _____

- How could you make use of these insights in the upcoming week?_____

  _____

Favorite remedies

Your health priorities will also guide your choice of self-care strategies. We all have our favorite personal treatments and we tend to rely on these first, no matter what health problems we face. We each have our own private stock of tried-and-true remedies for every health dilemma.

If physical exercise generally gets you out of a rut, you'll be likely to try exercise when your body feels tired, when you feel discouraged and empty, or when you can't concentrate very well. If talking with a friend generally helps you feel better, then you're likely to find a friend to talk with, whether your problem is a headache, or the inability to sleep, or loneliness. When you use your old favorites, they're likely to help—no matter what your problem really is. Why? Because you're comfortable with them, and they "turn you on" again.

The principle of wholeness indicates that the entirety of your health will probably be improved no matter which tried-and-true remedy you use. So go ahead and use your strengths whenever you can. Just don't limit yourself too narrowly. If your old favorites don't work, try something totally new.

How about you? What self-care remedies do you usually rely on to help you feel better?

Favorite Remedies Ranking

- Brainstorm some of the health remedies you use for improving your personal well-being. List at least five in each area.

Body	Mind	Relationships	Spirit
regular swimming	read a good book	cry with a friend	pray
massage	tell a joke	say thank you	watch the sunrise
_____	_____	_____	_____
_____	_____	_____	_____
_____	_____	_____	_____
_____	_____	_____	_____
_____	_____	_____	_____
_____	_____	_____	_____
_____	_____	_____	_____

- Go back and circle your favorite self-care remedies.

  Are they primarily physical, mental, relational, or spiritual? _____

- Which is your all-time favorite remedy, the one you fall back on when all else fails?

  _____

- Is your list different than it was five years ago or still essentially the same? _____

  In what ways? Why? _____

  _____

- Observations/insights/reflections on what you have written: _____

  _____

- How could you make use of these insights in the upcoming week? _____

  _____

Match the remedy to the symptom

If your "all-purpose" remedy doesn't work for a particular life situation, how do you make some other midcourse correction that might be more effective?

Most of us have trained ourselves to tackle problems head-on with logic. And the logical place to start would be to select the remedies most likely to relieve the symptoms of discomfort you're experiencing. Here are some of those logical self-care treatments.

For physical symptoms choose physical treatment—exercise; sleep; meditate; change eating, smoking, and drinking habits; use relaxation techniques; take medication; have surgery if necessary.

For mental symptoms choose mental treatment: accept yourself; talk with someone; try new behaviors; work on your fears; read; take a course; get more information; analyze your blocks; find new challenges.

For relational symptoms choose relational treatment: find new friends; smile more; give compliments; join an interest group; talk with a friend; reach out; love; trust.

For spiritual symptoms choose spiritual treatment: pray; meditate; accept doubts; confess; make a commitment; worship; reflect.

To be sure, the logical approach might lead to a successful strategy for enhancing your health. It's possible, however, that a remedy from a different life dimension would prove to be just as effective, or even more effective, than the most logical choice.

Or try a new combination

Since we are whole people, change in any dimension of well-being will affect our overall health. Any strategy we try has a good chance to help us. Could exercise help relieve your feelings of loneliness? Why not! Could prayer help you quit smoking? Maybe so. Check it out for yourself, combine any possible remedies with any symptom, and ask yourself, "Could it help?" You'll probably see that it could.

So if you have a problem—you're tired and run-down, or you're feeling pressure at work, or you're worried about a child, or you're depressed and feel empty, or you don't have many friends. What might help?

Starting an iron supplement?

Talking with someone who understands?

Taking your kids fishing?

Giving out compliments?

Instituting a lunch hour exercise program?

Writing in a journal?

Having an affair with your spouse?

Focusing on your spiritual development?

Calling an old friend?

Volunteering to coach Little League baseball?

Yes, yes, yes! These and thousands of other ideas might be just what you need.

Don't limit yourself to self-care strategies that make "sense." Search out new possibilities in every aspect of life. Try going back to school, or springboard diving, or values clarification, or time management, or square dancing, or a women's group, or evening devotions, or a vegetarian diet. Any of these could bring you renewed health and wholeness.

Since your self-care choices are unlimited, don't pick the dull ones. Pick the ones that turn you on. Choose some crazy, far-out ideas. If they make you laugh, that's great.

No matter what self-care strategy you choose, you can double its effectiveness by adding a creative twist, and you'll also double your enthusiasm for implementing the plan.

Creativity enhances any remedy

Beyond self-care

Conventional wisdom dictates that a book about wellness should end here. Most do. People often think of health as a private, personal matter. This book has already covered every aspect of self-care from body to mind to relationships to spirit. So why isn't this the end?

Why? Because taking care only of yourself—even taking care of your health in all dimensions—is too shallow a goal for true well-being. To stop with self-care could suggest that personal health is an end in itself, a goal for living. But that's not true!

To keep a healthy balance in your life, you need to go beyond self-absorption and ask yourself, "What am I going to do with my health? What's the purpose of all this self-care?" These questions will lead you beyond wellness to the deeper challenges of well-being—care for and commitment to others and investment of yourself in responsible work. Your personal well-being must be used to make a positive difference in your world. People who are truly whole and healthy reach out.

How can you reach out with a healthy commitment to others and to your work? The next chapters will help you tackle this question.

8

BEING WELL-to-DO

The reach-out dimension

Bored millionaires buy store

Sheffield, England

George and Elaine Dawes are buying a sporting goods store. They got bored at having nothing to do after winning a $1.8 million lottery jackpot.

"We don't want to be idle for the rest of our lives," George Dawes told reporters Sunday.

After their big win last year for guessing the results of soccer matches, the couple stopped working. George Dawes, 39, gave up his job as a salesman and his wife, 37, closed down her neighborhood general store.

They bought a luxury house with a swimming pool and a Rolls-Royce and took holidays in the Caribbean, the Mediterranean, and Europe.

"Now we are looking forward to getting up early in the morning once again," Elaine Dawes said.

Every one of us needs a reason to get up in the morning.

What's yours? You want to make something of yourself? You want to stack up enough money so that you and your family will be secure no matter what happens to the economy? You want the freedom to take exotic vacations? You want to be more successful than your neighbors and friends? If so, like this couple, one morning you're likely to wake up aching with emptiness. Money, freedom, fancy toys, and exotic vacations are not enough to sustain us day after day.

The power of purpose

We all need a reason, a purpose outside of ourselves, to get up in the morning. Taking care of our own needs, desires, and wishes won't sustain us for long. Good self-care habits give us the ability to respond to others. This response-ability must be exercised or it withers—and with it we shrivel too.

To be truly healthy we need to focus on people and purposes beyond ourselves. Service to people and causes outside ourselves gives us the energy for tackling another day. Responsible work gives us a reason to get up.

What about you? What are your responsibilities, your purposes, and your commitments like these days?

Purpose Assessment

- What are the main purposes and responsibilities that get you out of bed morning after morning? Your work? A project? Your children? A goal? Your desire to help others? Financial stability? _____

  _____

- In what kind of work are you investing yourself? _____

  _____

- To what outside of yourself are you committed? _____

  _____

- To whom have you committed yourself with care? _____

  _____

- What positive difference are you trying to make in your world? _____

  _____

The balance challenge

Even after we make commitments to our job and to our family and to others in our world, we still have to determine how we will split our time and energy between all these competing demands. Again, we are challenged to find a healthy balance.

It is difficult to find a healthy balance among all the possibilities to which you could give yourself. How do you choose to balance your time commitments to your kids, your spouse, your work, your parents, your church—and to the myriad of other responsibilities screaming for your attention? How do you balance the needs of one against the other and determine which is most important at the moment? How do you get your life back in balance when you find yourself pushed and pulled in too many directions at once?

These are tough questions. Finding a healthy balance between your various commitments is guaranteed to be a difficult and demanding task. Why?

Because unless you choose to become a hermit, there are always too many things to do, and too many people to pay attention to, and too little time in which to get it all done. Before we make any real commitments we have to make some decisions. With only a limited amount of time and energy, we can't commit ourselves to getting all our work done and responding to the needs of everyone we know and every cause that comes by. We must make choices—difficult choices.

Some people decide to find their outreach balance by giving a bit of themselves to many different possibilities—by trying to balance the demands of family, work, and others in reasonably equal proportions. Other people respond to the healthy balance challenge by focusing intensely on a smaller number of commitments. They may, for a period of years, focus primarily on their career, or on their family, or on a specific cause, while letting go of most other options. The healthy balance can take many different forms. Consider these examples.

Faith and Dorothy

Faith Nelson and Dorothy Hallen are cousins who have lived together as a family since early childhood. Until retirement, Dorothy was a dedicated elementary school teacher. Faith continues to teach young piano students.

They are devoted to each other but have made room in their lives for a circle of close friends and a wide variety of acquaintances. They participate in study groups. They volunteer many hours a week at their church. They gave years of their lives to care for an elderly friend. After his death they had the freedom to travel so they treated themselves to a trip to England.

Faith and Dorothy have lived balanced lives. Sometimes they gave more to work, other times to friends. Sometimes they postponed personal plans to help a neighbor. But over the years there has been a healthy balance in their lives. It didn't just happen. They made decisions about what was important, then they made sure that their day-to-day choices implemented those decisions.

Diane

Diane Anderson gives herself fully to her work. Every day she comes home exhausted, with a pile of work still left for the evenings. By the end of the week she needs the weekend just to catch up and regain her energy.

A compulsive workaholic? No! Diane is a high school English teacher. She knows that excellent communication skills are essential in today's world and she's committed to helping each of her students become as skillful as they can be. Her students' papers are returned with carefully thought out encouragement and suggestions, never just check marks or a grade.

She doesn't make as much money as some of her friends, but she loves her work, and her students often return to tell her that they sailed through their college papers with flying colors!

Patrick

Patrick Grant goes to college full-time and is responsible for paying his own tuition. He has to work night shifts at a convenience store to pay for everything. His studying and sleeping habits are getting much worse.

He has little time to make friends and to enjoy the college experience as he'd like, but he feels that these "extras" must be sacrificed so that he can graduate without a burdensome debt.

Paul and Sarah

Years ago Paul and Sarah Goodman made a commitment to keep their family life central. They shared the belief that parenting was a top priority and they discussed the issue with each other at length, even before marriage. As their four children have grown through adolescence, they have had to affirm and reaffirm their commitment to their family over and over again.

The Goodmans' investment in parenting has carried a high price tag. Over the years first Paul and later Sarah have each taken on stimulating careers. But the Goodmans have never allowed their careers to eat up family time. Family friendships take precedence over the pursuit of friendships that exclude children. Leisurely vacations as a couple have been replaced by hectic, inexpensive camping trips with the kids. Sleep, once lost for sick children, is now interrupted by calls from stranded kids or crack-of-dawn chauffeuring. Any extra money goes for musical instruments or the kids' education funds rather than for luxuries for parents. Do the Goodmans complain about the cost of this sacrifice? Absolutely not!

Like all parents, the Goodmans have no guarantee that their children will turn out the way they imagine and hope. Paul and Sarah know their limitations and affirm their own efforts: "We took our best shot at it. Now we'll just have to see."

Fred and Sue

Fred and Sue Morris made a commitment as well. Solid, midwestern beef-eaters, they chose to become vegetarians several years ago—not for food preference or health reasons, but on principle. "Since so much of the world is hungry," they reasoned, "we should eat lower on the food chain. If everyone did so, there would be enough food for all." Every day they pay for that decision. Neighbors and friends don't understand. Meal preparation takes more time. Eating out is almost impossible. And, what's more, they both still like meat.

Will the Morrises' commitment to this principle make the world a better place? Will it influence others? They hope so, but don't know. Fred and Sue accept the cost of their cause with no guarantees of success.

Evaluate your balance

No person is totally untouched by the challenge of balance, but most of us do find ways to do our jobs well, to reach out and touch others, and to take care of ourselves.

How well are you balancing your life these days? Take a moment to ponder your present priorities. The inventory below will help you analyze your current outreach patterns and the ways in which you are currently spending your time and energy. Check the statements which apply to you.

Reach-Out Inventory

Purpose/Commitment

___ I am clear about who I am, my purpose in life and my values.

___ I invest myself whole-heartedly in the present, rather than waiting around for my "real" life to begin.

___ I am committed to at least one project that will improve the quality of life for someone else.

___ I am clear enough about my priorities that I can say "no" when I need to.

___ I carefully consider my outside involvements so that I can fully commit myself to those in which I truly believe.

___ I feel a passion for some causes that are outside of me and are bigger than just my own self-interest.

Family/Friends

___ Staying in touch with my family is a top priority for me.

___ I readily accept the responsibility to care for dependent family members who are less able than I because of age, health, or abilities.

___ I have said "no" to stimulating life options in order to care for my family. For periods of time I have made the family's welfare more important than my own.

___ I accept and affirm each family member as he or she is, complete with strengths and weaknesses, beauty and blemishes.

___ I regularly participate in family time: special rituals, celebrations, and traditions that promote communication and a positive history.

___ I forgive my spouse (family, friends) readily and without resentment.

Neighbors/Community

___ I try to personally touch each person I meet each day with kindness and warmth.

___ I practice being attentive to the needs of others around me—even if those needs are unspoken. I'm willing to bear others' burdens in any way I can.

___ I am a good listener and can listen empathically without judgment.

___ I invest myself in building positive relationships and in building a strong and lasting set of friendships.

___ I volunteer to share my gifts for the good of others both in my close neighborhood and beyond.

___ I tell others what I appreciate about them.

Work/Service

___ Through my job I am able to utilize many of my best skills in the work that I do.

___ I feel satisfied with my current life-work.

___ My job meets most of my work-related needs.

___ I am committed to a cause beyond myself, and I invest some of my money, my time, and my energy in it.

___ I am compassionate and I speak up whenever anyone is put down because of their race, sex, or religious views.

___ Through my work and service I am contributing to making this world a better place.

Count up your check marks for each category and record them below

Family/Friends _____   Neighbors/Community _____

Work/Service   _____   Purpose/Commitment _____   TOTAL ____

■ How to interpret your score:

The total number of checks on your **Reach-Out Inventory** provides you with an indication of your investments in service and self-sacrifice. Compare your total score with the Healthy Balance standards:

20-24 Excellent: You're obviously intent on making a positive difference in your world.
14-19 Average: You do reach out, but you might consider expanding your reach.
Below 13 Poor: You're in danger of being self-engrossed.

Take a few minutes to reflect on your outreach score and your reactions to it. Use the worksheet below to record your insights and any resolutions for change.

Personal Reflections on My Well-To-Do Pattern

■ In which areas are my current outreach investments adequate?_____

_____

■ In which areas am I neglecting my responsibility? _____

_____

Note my reactions: _____

■ In which areas would I like to increase or decrease my investment of self? _____

_____

■ Which specific habits would I like to modify?_____

_____

For specifics on your outreach patterns, pay particular attention to your score in each of the four items: Purpose/ Commitment, Family/Friends, Neighbors/Community, and Work/Service. If you checked three or less items in any dimension you may be neglecting your responsibility to reach out in that area.

In those areas where you checked four or more items you're probably reaching out with an energy and commitment that allows you to make a positive difference in your world.

Make healthful investments

Commitment to service that focuses on giving rather than receiving, characterized by the repeated choice to reach out and love, is an essential element in well-being. You cannot be well unless you reach out. Whole people are well-to-do. They reach out to the people around them and they invest themselves and their skills in meaningful work and service.

The next three chapters will focus specifically on the three outreach dimensions: your care for those closest to you; your outreach to neighbors in your community; and your commitment to your life-work.

As you explore your options for reaching out in the next three chapters, affirm your strengths and focus on those areas where you'd like to improve. Then share your reactions with someone you love.

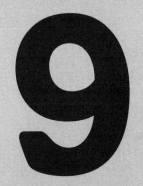

9

CARING for YOUR FAMILY

Reach out to the people close to you

Most of us learn our major lessons about relationships in the context of our families. At its best, the family offers us the most intense opportunity to give and to receive emotional support. At its worst, it confronts us with the risk of experiencing pain and distrust. In both cases, the family provides us with the crucible for learning to reach out with care, despite the possible costs.

Reach out to your family

Commitment is the glue that holds families together. The repeated decision to stick together through the best and worst of times, to care for one another, and to sacrifice when necessary for the common good—these commitments are the essence of family, and they make the family a valuable health resource for its members.

Commitment to family takes effort on our part, and requires an intense investment.

In our first family our parents took care of us, but for most of us as we grow into adulthood the care-giving changes direction. Suddenly we become the nurturers rather than the nurtured. Our attention shifts from having our needs met to putting the needs of others first.

Now, each time we choose to care for our family, even when we don't really feel like it, we forfeit the immediate rewards of self-gratification in favor of the long-term gains of intimacy and commitment.

Self-denial and self-sacrifice come with the territory. You sacrifice for your children, for your parents, for your partner. You offer whatever is needed regardless of the cost because you believe that the other person's welfare is equally important and sometimes even more important than your own. What parent wouldn't sacrifice a night's sleep to care for a sick child?

This kind of reaching out in commitment to family is essential to well-being. As we give ourselves to others, we grow in caring, tolerance, and understanding.

Here are three tips for enhancing the quality of your outreach to your family.

Tips for family outreach

Make the family top priority. The healthiest families have one characteristic in common: they make deliberate decisions to invest time and energy in their relationships with each other. They make family a number one priority.

Keeping the family as a top priority helps us decide how to invest our limited resources. When the children are still at home, that's the time to choose outside activities that include the family: be a Scout leader or work with the PTA, plan family outings and activities, connect with other families whose children mesh with yours. Later in life you'll have time to involve yourself elsewhere. If you throw yourself into too many activities away from home, you may not have the reserves you will need to deal with all the predictable and unpredictable crises that will come along.

Healthy outreach also extends beyond the boundaries of the nuclear family. Including Grandma in your outing to the 4th of July parade or to a piano recital affirms your commitment to family. So what if she dresses in strange clothing and talks too loudly—she's still family! Spending the weekend with your brother and his family, even when few of your needs get met in the interaction, can be a healthy outreach as well.

And if blood relatives aren't available or receptive, adopt

some "soul relatives" as your family and reach out to them. Remember, you make family by investing in deep, long-term relationships. Create your own family by reaching out intensely with a few people.

There's something intrinsically healthy about being part of a family and staying in touch with its multiple generations. Make family a top priority.

What about you? What level of priority have you made your family?

Family Priority Assessment

■ How much of your time and energy do you invest in your family? _____%

What sacrifices do you make to honor these commitments?_____

What healthy benefits do you receive? _____

■ Where does family fit in your priorities? _____

Are there any family members with whom you need to mend fences? _____

Who?_____

Find the forgiveness factor. What happens in a family when problems don't get solved? When people are angry with one another? Or envious? When people hurt or misunderstand each other?

Families need some way to reach out to one another with love and forgiveness. Most of us haven't had much experience with true forgiveness. We need to learn how to ask for, grant, and accept forgiveness.

Where do you start? How do you give and receive forgiveness in your family?

The starting point is to acknowledge that forgiveness is not a feeling, it's a choice. It's actually two choices—the decision made by one person to repent and the decision made by the other to forgive. When you've done something for which you need forgiveness, admit it. Swallow your pride, take the risk, and make your request directly: "Will you forgive me?"

Because we live so closely together in the family, our relationships at times are punctuated by conflict and accented by strong feeling. How do we build bridges in place of walls? How do we repair broken promises? How do we rebuild trust? How do we heal violated relationships? Every family needs mechanisms for forgiveness so that it can start over fresh—again and again. A note, the gift of a flower, a special favor—seek out and practice a variety of rituals for asking and offering forgiveness in your family.

What about you? Have you found ways for forgiveness to be expressed in your family?

Family Forgiveness Factor

- What's the forgiveness factor like in your family?

  Describe how it usually works. _____

  _____

  Which transgressions are the hardest for you to forgive? _____

  _____

  In what ways do you avoid asking for or offering direct forgiveness? _____

  _____

  What forgiveness rituals might work well for you? _____

  _____

Accentuate the positive. It's all too easy to get caught in the habit of being critical and judgmental of others, especially those in your family.

Why not focus on what you appreciate about the members of your family? The most wonderful gift we can give to one another is affirmation. So, say, "I love you." Don't delegate this powerful gift. Don't assume that others know you care.

Affirm one another. Focus on your family, and identify several qualities that make each family member unique. Tell each what you appreciate as special about him or her.

What about you? Does each person in your family feel special?

Family Affirmation Assessment

■ How positive are you in your family?

In what ways do you focus on being positive in your family? _____

_____

In what instances do you find yourself being quite critical and negative?_____

_____

What would you like to improve on? _____

_____

■ Observations/insights/comments on your outreach to family: _____

_____

_____

_____

The family is our most intense context for practicing the healthy art of reaching out to care for others. Although the costs of sacrifice may at times seem to outweigh the rewards, your investment of yourself over time will bring you a richness and depth found no other way.

Reach out to your partner

While some people are married and some are not, the struggles and principles discussed here are relevant to any deep, long-term, committed relationship. So, whether or not you're currently married as you read these suggestions, test them out against your own life experiences.

Any time we make a long-term commitment to another person we do so with positive expectations that the relationship will be fulfilling, joyful—maybe even "happily ever after." That's not a bad way to start a serious relationship—full of hope.

But it's a rare couple who is able to pull off the happily ever after part. Marriage as a lifelong relationship usually doesn't go quite that smoothly. It doesn't take couples long to find out that two don't become one without some difficulties.

If your expectations coincide with those of your spouse, there's no problem. When they differ, watch out! Misunderstandings, hurt feelings, and anger are just around the corner. The "happily ever after" suddenly may not be very happy, and you may wonder if it will last forever.

Whenever problems occur, you must roll up your sleeves and get down to work. Marriages are not made in heaven. They don't just happen. People make them happen by the choices and sacrifices they make over the years. Marriages that last are based on hard work and a large measure of caring commitment.

Here are four tips for enhancing the quality of your relationship with your spouse.

Tips for a healthy marriage

Keep in touch with each other. The key to the health of any loving relationship is communication. Marriage is no exception. If you want to maintain a strong and vibrant relationship, you need to talk with each other regularly and openly about your commitment and the issues that affect it. Marriage requires attention and maintenance to weather life's storms. Listening and sharing in a positive caring atmosphere enhances the well-being of both parties.

Marriage Relationship Assessment

■ What hassles and trivia currently get in the way of your keeping in touch with each other?

_____

_____

■ How could you plan to put those items aside for a time and really focus on each other?

_____

_____

■ How could you renew your covenant? _____

_____

_____

Renew your covenant. Regularly renew your promises and your commitment to each other. The Old Testament uses the word "covenant" to describe the special promises and commitments that bind husband and wife together. The concept of covenant seems particulary appropriate when talking about marriage, since it suggests depth, permanence, dialog, and wholeness.

Covenants are more than agreements about who walks the dog and how towels get folded. A covenant is a sacred promise—a pledge of commitment. The promises implicit in a covenant include cherishing one another, respecting one another fully, putting the other's welfare ahead of your own, forgiving, and choosing to love in ways that transcend the day-to-day inconveniences, petty annoyances, and disappointments of living under the same roof year after year.

Marriage Reaffirmation Assessment

- In what ways have you and your partner reaffirmed and adapted your marriage covenant over the past few years?_____

  _____

- How could you make the process of nurturing your commitment more intentional and meaningful? _____

  _____

  _____

- How could you accept the limits of your relationship? _____

  _____

  _____

Accept the limits of your relationship. Every relationship has areas of chronic trouble. They're called chronic because they just won't go away. Rather than continue to ask, "How can I get rid of this?" or "How can I change my spouse?" you might be better off asking, "How can I learn to live with this difficulty?"

It's not so awful to experience chronic problems. They may be painful, but pain is a part of life. They may cause you to be lonely, but it's possible to live with some loneliness. It's OK to have a less-than-perfect relationship! Too many people get trapped into ending a good thing just because it's not perfect.

Don't sell yourself a bill of goods. Your relationship does not have to be perfect to be loving.

Both your personal depth and the strength of your commitment are enhanced by your toughest thorns. You do grow and mature in response to difficulties. Every problem is a teacher. Allow those difficulties that won't go away to be your instructors for life—and to deepen your relationship.

Marriage Problem Assessment

- List a couple of the limitations/chronic problems/irreconcilable differences in your relationship.

  _____

- What have these problems taught you?

  About yourself? _____

  About life? _____

  About commitment? _____

- If you were to quit trying to change the problems and learn to accept them as chronic, what positive direction would you then be freed to focus on?_____

  _____

Accept imbalance in the giving/getting ratio. As with all commitments, "hanging in there" in marriage over the years requires self-denial and self-sacrifice. At some points your own self-fulfillment will be curtailed, at least in the short run.

Marriage is not always a 50–50 proposition. Much of the time it's an 80–20 affair, with partners alternating the responsibility for energy investment. In some relationships the 80–20 is always weighted in the same direction. During some periods, especially in a crisis, one of you may be giving 100 percent while the other is unwilling, or unable, to give much at all. At other times your relationship may be 35–35 with both of you investing less than your fair share. Occasionally you may find that both of you pour your heart and soul into your relationship at an 80–80 clip.

Marriage gives us a structure for self-sacrifice in depth. Marriages that work are based on the choices made over the years to reach out and care for each other's welfare whatever the cost.

Commitment provides the glue for a relationship that holds you and your spouse together when your relationship seems way out of balance.

How about you?

Marriage Balance Assessment

- What percent are you giving and getting in your relationship these days?

  I am giving _____ %   My partner is giving _____ %

  I am getting _____ %   My partner is getting _____ %

- What would you like to see improved? _____

  _____

Talk your answers over with your spouse. Notice the issues you agree on and those you don't. Remember: listen carefully —don't accuse!

Marriage can (and for many people does) become the most intense experiment in reaching out to another human being with a mixture of commitment and depth, uncertainty and pain, intimacy and joy.

In the next chapter you will look at your patterns for reaching out to your friends and neighbors. But first, stop for a moment and consider your current commitments to your family and your partner.

Personal Reflection on My Outreach to Family and Spouse

■ The priority I give to family _____

_____

■ The time and energy I am currently investing in my family _____

_____

■ The forgiveness factor in my family _____

_____

■ The affirmation I offer to family members _____

_____

■ The problem solving patterns in my family _____

_____

■ What, if anything would I like to change _____

_____

_____

Wish List for Health-Fullness in My Family

■ List here everything you can imagine wanting in your outreach to your family. What would you like to be able to do? To feel? Let your imagination run free. Don't limit yourself in any way. The wishes don't have to be practical.

I wish I could: _____

_____

_____

_____

_____

10

CARING for OTHERS

Reach out to the people around you

Most of us practice our skills at reaching out with care to others most intensely within the context of our families. But our commitments to outreach must also extend beyond the boundaries of family.

Well-being is enhanced by a commitment to care for others that focuses on giving rather than receiving and that repeatedly chooses to reach out in love to whichever neighbor needs us at the moment. As you read this chapter about the problems and possibilities for reaching out to your wider range of neighbors, reflect on the balance of caring commitments in your life.

Reach out to your neighbors

Reaching out can be a risky business. When you commit yourself to loving your neighbor in general, you never know when a particular neighbor is going to pop up with a need you can fill. It takes an attitude of openness and curiosity to leave your personal circle of security and step across invisible boundaries into the unknown.

It's not too hard to offer your services to an elderly neighbor whose lawn needs mowing. Or to a friend who needs a ride to the dentist. You may gladly volunteer for a chamber of commerce committee or cancel a movie date to spend the evening visiting an acquaintance who's hospitalized. The risk of reaching out to people in our own circle is minimal. But most of us draw that circle quite tightly around ourselves and thereby close ourselves off from a world full of neighbors.

Think of the last party you went to, or church potluck, or school meeting. Which people did you include in your reach-out circle? Which did you ignore or interact with only superficially? For most of us the second group is by far the larger.

What about all the people you know only by face—bus drivers, salespeople, old folks, shopkeepers, airline attendants? Are you businesslike and formal with them, or even rude when they don't jump to meet your needs?

The neat, clean lines we're tempted to draw between the people who belong in our neighborhood and receive our care, and those who don't belong and are therefore excluded from our care-giving, tend to disappear in times of crisis when our connections as part of the human family suddenly, unexpectedly, draw us closely together in intimate contact with strangers.

People need people. And reaching out with care and concern for another heals both the receiver and the giver! Break beyond your boundaries and give yourself to others. They need you.

The investment will take energy. Your focus on others may drain you. It will certainly take time from your private pursuits. You'll risk rebuff and rejection. You'll experience loss and grief when neighbors you have loved die or go away. The rewards are uncertain. But it's worth the risk. You can't be truly well in isolation. Reach out. Choose to love.

You can make a difference in your world by reaching out with your attitudes, with your heart, with your hands, and with thanksgiving. Check yourself and your reach-out habits against the following suggestions.

Reach out with your attitude

Choose an attitude that opens your heart to let people in, rather than closing your heart to keep people out. Easier said than done.

It's so much simpler to base our judgments about others on very little information—physical appearance, the tone of voice, clothing, age. We decide this person is a snob. That one is spacey. Another is a rigid conservative. In our minds we draw a circle that includes some and excludes others. All these judgments are based on our attitudes.

Have you ever been thrown together with someone you had previously locked out of your circle and soon discovered, much to your surprise, that as you got to know that person better you found that he or she was intriguing? Did your opinion about this person change, and did you allow him or her to enter your circle? If so, your neighborhood was enlarged with just a simple change in attitude!

The real test of our capacity to reach out in a health enhancing manner comes when we consider the people we tend to write off and write out of our lives—the undesirables, the unloved, the forgotten. Remember, this list may include spouse or family as well!

Most of us structure our lives so that we aren't confronted by the needs of those fellow human beings who make us uncomfortable, who evoke from us an involuntary shudder or a nervous laugh. Yet these people are also the neighbors we are called to serve, no matter how we feel at the time.

How about you? Are you reaching out to a wide variety of people, both acquaintances and strangers?

Attitude Assessment

■ What types of people never or rarely have the opportunity to experience your care for them? People who have physical defects? Different skin color? Strange language? Mental limitations? People who are ill? Odd? Old? Fragile? Disoriented? Deaf? Crazy? People who make you angry? Frighten you? Repulse you? Who are they?

_____, _____, _____,

_____, _____, _____

■ Stretch your attitude. Think about the week ahead and the people you're likely to make contact with at home, work, shopping, church, meetings, concerts. Name one person you would usually brush past or greet only perfunctorily—a bank teller, a construction worker, your principal, a crotchety neighbor, the blind woman who rides your bus, the Vietnam vet in the next office.
Name:_____

■ Focus on that person now for a minute. Open your mind and consider what that individual might be like as a human being.

What needs might this neighbor be carrying that you could meet?_____

_____

What might brighten the day for this person? _____

_____

What could you do to reach out?_____

_____

■ Resolve to reach out and make positive contact with this neighbor at your next opportunity. Use some of the ideas in the rest of this chapter. See what happens. Work to expand this attitude of openness to more and more people.

My resolve:_____

_____

The call to service and self-sacrifice challenges us to respect and respond to the humanness of each person, from close family, to bosom buddy, to street person. People who reach out regularly evidence a deep respect for others as people. They offer an outlook of positive expectation to strangers as well as friends, to check-out clerks as well as colleagues, to waitresses as well as tennis partners.

Compassion and gentleness in day-to-day living requires that an attitude of openness, curiosity, and caring pervade all our human contact.

Reach out with your heart

The most valuable skill for reaching out to others is the art of listening with your heart. This gift of listening deeply and carefully to the concerns and feelings of another person is called empathy.

Empathy literally means to "feel in"—to stand in another's shoes for a moment, to get inside another person's feelings. Through the process of tuning in to another's feelings and responding in a way that confirms what you have heard, you can show understanding and acceptance.

Everyone needs empathy.

Look around at the signals your neighbors are sending. What about the troublemaker in your son's homeroom? Do you suppose he could be saying, "No one knows how I feel. No one cares."? What about the person who pushes ahead of you in line at the post office. Is it possible she needs someone to listen to the pain in her life? What about your colleague who's always putting other people down. Could she really be asking, "Please, someone understand me!" What about your spouse? Is your partner hoping that you show signs that you care? Or what about your mother who may be feeling lonely and left out? Or your son who is worried about whether or not he'll succeed? Everyone aches to be understood fully and to have their feelings accepted. The signs are all around us!

Empathy is hard work. You have to pay attention—yes, pay! It costs something when you choose to tune in to someone else. It takes time, energy, and the determinaton to focus on meeting another person's needs rather than your own.

The sharing, understanding, and accepting of feelings form the heart of human relationships. Empathy is the skill that activates these processes between people and allows people to give themselves to each other.

How about you? What kind of listener are you?

Listening Assessment

■ When was the last time you gave your full attention as a gift to someone else, and really listened closely?_____

■ Think back over today. What bad listening habits prevented you from listening with your heart? The situation?_____

What stopped you from hearing the feelings? Fear of yourself? Wanting to fix the problem? Afraid of the results? Asking too many questions? Disagreement with what the person was saying? The desire to give advice? Focusing on your own problems? Wanting to be liked?

What stopped you? _____

Thinking about that situation now, how could you have listened more carefully?

_____

What positive effect do you imagine that listening would have had on the conversation? On the other person? _____

_____

True listening is rare. It is a gift of yourself you can give to another. We have two eyes to see with, two ears to hear with, two nostrils to smell with, and two hands to touch with; but only one mouth to talk with—and we use that much more than we should! Since we have two ears, we should listen at least twice as much as we talk.

How could you practice listening more fully? With what neighbors will you start? Reach out and touch someone with your eyes, your ears, and your heart. Show that you care. Listen!

Reach out with your hands

Reach out and touch someone—really touch someone. Does that suggestion raise the hair on the back of your neck? Frighten you? Perhaps even excite you? As we were growing up, most of us learned to keep our hands to ourselves and not to invade other people's space. We learned our lesson so well that when we bump into someone in a crowded elevator we say "Excuse me," rather than "You're welcome!" In this society we keep our distance.

How sad! Physical contact is one of life's richest blessings—a powerful means of communication and a largely neglected health-giving resource.

Why not get used to giving people hugs. It's not that hard. Some people may be surprised at first, but if you practice it often enough, your neighbors will soon figure out you're for real. Don't be surprised if they start hanging around you, waiting for more of the same.

Touch is a powerful way to reach out. Are you offering and receiving its benefits?

Physical Closeness Assessment

- How do you feel when people touch you? _____

  _____

- How much is physical closeness and touching a regular part of your daily life outside the family? _____

  _____

- What are your rules about touching? _____

  _____

- Who needs to be touched by you today?_____, _____

  _____, _____, _____

Positive caring demonstrated by physical contact lets high energy flow between people, filling each person with vigor and vitality. You can hardly touch without being touched in return. You have a marvelous health-giving resource at the end of your arms and many touch-hungry neighbors waiting for physical strokes. Initiate a health-enhancing exchange. Make sure that touch is a part of every contact you make.

Reach out with thanksgiving

A little appreciation goes a long, long way. Studies have shown that gratitude is a more powerful motivator than money. Most of us will really put ourselves out just to hear someone say, "Thank you."

When a friend or a stranger reaches out to you, returning the gift in kind is rarely necessary. Usually a simple sign that you appreciate the kindness will be gift enough. Gratitude is a way of reaching out in return.

If you want to improve your thanks-giving style, you could try one or more of these suggestions.

Form a mutual-admiration group. If some people in your life don't like to give and receive appreciation, find some who do and spend time with them.

Select small, unique gifts that carry a personal message from your heart. Surprise people with them. Gifts you create— poems, notes, wall hangings—speak most clearly.

Once again, get into the habit of thanks-giving. Say it directly! "Thanks for listening to me." "You're always so positive. Thanks!" "Knowing you care keeps me going. Thanks!"

Thanks-giving Assessment

■ How do you feel when someone tells you directly how much they appreciate you?

_____

_____

■ In what ways do you reach out to others by showing gratitude? _____

_____

■ In what ways are you careless about remembering to demonstrate your appreciation?

_____

_____

■ Who needs to hear a "thank you" from you today?

_____ , _____ , _____

_____ , _____ , _____

To be truly healthy we must reach out beyond ourselves. Make friends. Give support. Pay attention to the needs of others. Encourage others to take care of themselves. Whenever we offer acceptance, love, forgiveness, or a quiet word of hope, we offer health. When we share each other's burdens and joys, we become channels of healing. No matter how timid or tired or selfish or crazy or young or old we are, we all have something important to offer each other.

Your neighbors need your support and care. To offer yourself is a choice you alone can make. Love is a decision, not a feeling. If you want to promote love, live like a lover. You can choose to reach out and touch someone—many someones!

The trick in reaching out is to train yourself to notice others' needs and then be ready to share your gifts when they are appropriate.

Be prepared. You never know when your neighbor might need you. Where you see the need, step in and try to respond. Whenever you reach out to another, your own well-being is enhanced along with the well-being of the person who receives your care and concern.

How about you?

Before moving to the next chapter's focus, your commitment to investing yourself in meaningful life-work, stop for a moment and consider your current patterns of care-giving to the friends and neighbors around you.

Personal Reflection on My Outreach to Others

- My attitude toward people _____
  _____

- My listening skills _____
  _____

- My use of touch _____
  _____

- My actions of gratitude _____
  _____

- Am I satisfied with my outreach patterns? _____
  _____

- What, if anything, would I like to change? _____
  _____

Wish List for My Health-Full Outreach

- List here everything you can imagine wanting in your outreach to others. What would you like to be able to do? To feel? Let your imagination run free. Don't limit yourself in any way. The wishes don't have to be practical.

  I wish I could: _____

  _____

  _____

  _____

  _____

11

INVESTING in MEANINGFUL WORK

Reach out to your world

If we want to be truly well, we can't limit our reaching out only to family and friends. We need also to invest ourselves responsibly in meaningful, productive work and service to the wider community. It's part of being an adult!

Work can be any activity that requires the investment of our time and energy. Work, whether for pay or not for pay, becomes for us yet another way of making a positive difference in our world.

Identify your work

Most of us in the "real world" have a job to support ourselves. And we think of it as a necessity, not as a chance to improve the world around us. Realistically, for most of us, holding a job is a necessity! But in spite of the fact that most jobs take eight hours per day, five days per week, and require from us a substantial commitment and responsibility, they also offer us the opportunity to utilize our skills and to invest our efforts in meaningful, productive activity.

Deep down inside we all enjoy being useful and effective. It's rewarding to see that we can create, accomplish tasks, and contribute our skills—that we can make a positive difference. For those of us without a paying job, the challenge is still the same—to find a life-work, a mission, in which we can believe; to find a way of being effective that brings us satisfaction.

If we are fortunate, our job allows us to do something beneficial that we believe in, and we feel proud of our accomplishments.

However, the overlap between "what must be done" and what "feels meaningful" is never 100%. Every job, every life, has its downside—tasks we must manage even though they bring us no particular meaning or joy.

Work Assessment

■ What work do you currently invest yourself in? (You may list many: job, school, family, household management, volunteer work, causes, dreams.) _____

_____

■ In what way does this work allow you to invest your skills meaningfully in a way that brings you joy and pride?_____

■ What difference do you hope to make through your work?

_____

_____

The energy and time that work requires may lead to exhaustion, frustration, and anger. These feelings are often experienced by those who follow a career path and who invest everything they have in their jobs. They're just as common for those who are employed at one job for money and who return home to another job—managing the house, cooking, caring for children or husbands—doing whatever is needed for whomever needs it. And they're felt just as frequently by those whose work involves multiple responsibilities at home or in the community but does not include the exchange of money.

Like caring for others, work is a commitment, with a risk and a cost. It's exhausting. So, don't be surprised when you see the signs of stress fatigue in yourself and others—because you will.

The stress of work

Many people feel under stress a good share of the time. In an informal survey a remarkable percentage of people in different professions reported that they are usually or always under stress: 80% of executives and managers, 66% of teachers and secretaries, 67% of farmers, and 61% of homemakers.

It's difficult and challenging to balance self-care, and reaching out to family and friends, along with the many responsibilities and jobs we each must accomplish each day. Sometimes it seems impossible! That's why finding the healthy balance, especially related to work, is often so difficult. There's simply too much to do, and not enough hours in the day to get it all done.

If work contributes to your unhealthy balance you may need to go back to your basic values and ask yourself whether or not you are spending too much of yourself on making money, and investing too little on yourself, your family, and your friends.

Why work?

Why do you work? For survival? For personal challenge? To upgrade your lifestyle? For the social contact? For the paycheck? For intellectual stimulation? To save for college tuition? What do you hope to give and receive as you invest yourself in your job?

Each of us wants something different from our work. Most of us, however, don't have a very clear idea about what motivates us to keep working day after day. It is important to clarify just what needs we expect our work to fulfill.

No one job can ever meet all of our needs. But for a job to be fulfilling, it must meet some of the basic needs that you

154

consider essential. When a job doesn't satisfy some of your key needs, it drains you rather than energizes you.

What you want out of your job may change. As you grow as a person, as you gain confidence or competence, as your life situation shifts, as the nature of your work changes, you may find different needs taking priority—and you may discover that your job has become more or less satisfying than before.

Your commitments may change. As your financial needs, family situation, age, and skill level are altered, your work related investments can and should change accordingly.

Job satisfaction contributes to well-being. Most of us spend a large part of the day working. Our work has a big impact on how we feel. When we can see that our efforts are making a significant contribution to something we believe in, we feel successful.

Jobs provide a complex mixture of rewards. There are many reasons for working. Although nearly everyone is motivated in part by the rewards of the "employee benefit package" (wages, insurance, pension, vacation, etc.), many other human needs are fulfilled by our work.

What about you? Is your life-work satisfying? Consider the twelve job motivators outlined below to discover your keys to effective performance and fulfillment. Then answer the questions in the worksheet.

12 reasons to work

Employment Package. To have enough money for your lifestyle, family, and future; to get ahead financially; to be safe and insured for unexpected emergencies or crises.

Variety. To have a change of pace from your personal and home life; to have a balance and regular hours and schedules; to experience true separation between work and home.

Positive Environment. To have a pleasant work environment, conducive to physical and mental health; to be located in a desirable area; to experience beauty.

Sense of Worth. To feel good about yourself; to experience confidence and personal power.

Affirmation. To receive recognition for your work; to be seen as highly skilled; to be looked up to with respect.

Relationships. To meet a variety of new people; to be accepted; to feel care from others and for them as well; to experience camaraderie and a sense of belonging.

Connection. To experience being part of a team; to be part of an organization of which you are proud; to know you are an important part of the whole.

Control. To have freedom to organize your work as you see best; to be responsible for specific decisions.

Productivity. To have an opportunity to be creative; to make something; to make up something; to make something happen; to accomplish something; to be productive; to solve problems.

Stimulation. To add excitement and adventure; to push yourself to grow and advance; to develop yourself and your skills.

Usefulness. To use your talents effectively; to match well with your interests, skills, and abilities.

Purpose. To give meaning to your life; to help others and make the world a better place; to grow in depth and understanding of the world and your place in it.

Work Motivation Assessment

- Identify some of the main reasons why you invest yourself in work and some of the rewards that you hope to receive. List your top priorities. What conditions in a job are absolutely essential to you? _____

  _____

  _____

- On a scale of 1 to 10 rank your current job against the standards of your "perfect" job.

  1 = My current job gives me nothing I want; 10 = I'm totally fulfilled in my current job

  1   2   3   4   5   6   7   8   9   10

- How has the fulfillment, or lack of fulfillment, of work-related needs affected your sense of well-being and satisfaction with your work? _____

  _____

  _____

- In what ways does your present job allow you to contribute of yourself? _____

  _____

  _____

- What challenge or opportunity to serve are you missing in your life these days?

  _____

  _____

Unfortunately, some jobs offer a paycheck but few opportunities for real fulfillment. They may be stressful, or boring, or without potential for advancement. Creativity may be stifled and supportive relationships discouraged.

If you'd like to make your investment in your work more fulfilling, consider implementing some of the suggestions below.

Make work more fulfilling

Alter your job so that it fulfills more of your needs. This may not be easy, and you may not have total control, but often you can make small changes—sometimes without anyone else even noticing—that will significantly enhance your job satisfaction.

Decide that you're getting enough satisfaction from your job right now! Accept it as it is. No job is perfect. Don't spend your life grumbling about minor irritants in your job if it is, in fact, giving you a large measure of fulfillment.

Look for the fulfillment of some unmet job needs through your personal life. Too much of this strategy might be dangerous, but sometimes you can take the edge off your frustration on the job by getting some of your needs met outside the work setting. For example, if relationships in your work environment are characterized by conflict, make sure that you build supportive friendships outside your work world.

Find fulfillment for your unmet job needs through volunteer work. If your job doesn't give you the chance to contribute in a way that you want, tackle a position in the community that will. For example, if your daily work isn't challenging enough, volunteer for a task that stretches your skills. Or if your job doesn't allow for much creativity, find a community project that requires dreaming and vision.

Look for another job that will be more fulfilling and rewarding for you. Yes, if you've discovered during this reflection process that your job is simply not fulfilling enough, a career change may be in order. You might want to start looking for something else that will be more motivating. You can't just thumb your nose at the security you have in your current job, but you do have the right to expect a lot more than just money when you invest yourself in your work—you have a right to expect that you can make a positive contribution.

You may, however, find that the very best of you, your imagination, creativity, sensitivity, and compassion, will best be expressed away from your job. You may do your most exciting work as a volunteer rather than for pay.

Consider how you might reach out to others and in doing so find deep satisfaction yourself.

Missions beyond work

A healthy balance also involves reaching out with compassion and concern for the "things" of creation and the people beyond our neighborhood. This reaching out must often be accomplished outside of our "real" jobs.

It is important to view ourselves as citizens of the worldwide community, called to responsibility for all creation. What an awesome undertaking! How does one start looking after the world? It's somewhat like eating an elephant: you just take one bite at a time.

The task begins with commitment, and involves sacrifice and risk-taking in the simple day-to-day choices about where we invest ourselves. These choices add up over time to create a solid commitment.

Consider these examples of people who have found their life mission outside of their work.

Alan Paton

South African Alan Paton, author of **Cry, the Beloved Country**, prominent spokesman for equality and justice, did not set out to be a crusader. Until middle age he was a reform-school administrator with little public visibility. In his writing, however, he responded to the cries of injustice he saw around him, and he spoke eloquently of the human cost of apartheid. As he matured, his moral commitments grew with him. Without seeking the role, he became an intellectual and spiritual leader, loved the world over but kept under surveillance in his own country.

Andy

A little closer to home, Andy started by talking to a wheelchair-bound classmate. Casual conversation led to genuine concern about the obstacles she faced in her effort to lead a normal life. Soon he was launched on a full-scale investigation into the needs of those unable to walk. Eventually Andy organized a student-interest group that lobbied effectively with the school board to allocate funds for several small changes that made life much easier for the handicapped students at his school. Andy went on to study architecture and now specializes in designing structures that enhance the lives of people with physical disabilities. A career of outreach and service began with a brief conversation and grew slowly over time with increasing levels of commitment.

Julie

Julie's decision to boycott a major food producer started with a movie at church about infant malnutrition in the Third World. She first learned about world hunger from a student distributing leaflets at the state fair. What she heard appalled her. Now she dines one night a week on the average diet of the less fortunate—one cup of rice—and she sends the money she saves to Bread for the World.

The Swansons took in a runaway for a weekend and discovered new purpose in life. Now they're part of a network of treatment homes for adolescents who desperately need loving structure.

The Swansons

Alan, Andy, Julie, and the Swansons—each of these people found new meaning and fuller health when they took that first small step to reach out and make a difference in their world.

How do we decide where to invest ourselves? It's tough! We have only a certain amount of personal resources—time, energy, and finances. The needs of creation are overwhelming. Should we tackle sudden infant death? Job discrimination? Illiteracy? Juvenile delinquency? Violence on TV? Violence between nations? Even if we do, will our efforts make any difference? Should we contribute to the Salvation Army? Public radio? Planned Parenthood? Cancer research? Foreign missions? Which causes truly deserve our attention and investment? It's a question of personal choice, based on personal values.

What about you? How do you respond to the needs of others?

Response to Human Needs Assessment

- What human problems concern you the most? _____

  _____

- Where have you chosen to commit yourself and your resources? _____

  _____

- What small steps have you aleady taken? (Start with the needs evident right in your own backyard and see where they lead you). _____

  _____

- What difference do you hope to make later in your life when you have more time?

  _____

  _____

The healthiest, most vital people are alert to situations in which they can help. They work efficiently, energetically, and effectively. They're always reaching out, looking for opportunities to care for their wold. They've discovered a secret many of us miss—the gift we give comes back to us, multiplied many times. When you reach out through your job or non-job activities, you open yourself to the healing experience of unity with all creation.

So reach out beyond yourself and the boundaries of your own immediate desires.

Before returning to the wider question of **Seeking Your Healthy Balance**, reflect on your pattern of reaching out to the world through your work and your service commitments. Do your reach-out habits in this area enhance your well-being? How do your habits affect the planet and its people?

Personal Reflection on My Outreach to the World

- The work that I do to utilize my skills _____

_____

- My sense of satisfaction and pride in my job _____

_____

- My commitment to principles (social justice, human rights, education) _____

_____

- My investment of time, energy, and resources in caring for creation (actions supporting wider causes and concerns) _____

_____

- What if anything I would like to change? _____

_____

_____

Wish List for Health-fullness in My Work

- List here everything you can imagine wanting to do in your work. The positive differences you would like to make, the abilities to reach out that you would like to develop. List your dreams about how you can influence your world for the better. Let your imaagination run free. The wishes don't have to be practical. Have fun dreaming.

  I wish I could: _____

  _____

  _____

  _____

  _____

12 RECOGNIZING UNHEALTHY PATTERNS

The healthy balance revisited

You can't be healthy unless you care for yourself. You aren't really healthy unless you put your health to good use—in meaningful work and in helping others. So there you have it again—the healthy balance dilemma

The healthy balance dilemma

On the one hand, well-being requires self-care—taking the best possible care of your body, mind, spirit—with all your strengths, limitations, potentials, and frailties. On the other hand, you can't be truly healthy without reaching out in service to meet the needs of others—nurturing your family; bearing another's burdens, listening to cries of pain, or despair, or anxiety; protecting your environment; and making a contribution to your world with your labor. When one aspect of health is pursued and worshiped as if it were the whole, the balance is upset and well-being will soon be forfeited.

This balance may look easy on paper, but it's never easy to practice. Why? Because there are no clear rules for determining when to do what.

The healthy balance is excruciatingly difficult to put into practice because at every moment you must be asking yourself, "Who and what should I be caring for now? Is now the time for me to work? Or to take care of myself? Or to care for you?"

When and under what circumstances do you neglect your own needs to take care of others first? Or neglect your work to take care of yourself? How do you decide?

It would be much more comfortable to latch on to one set of answers and relieve yourself of the decision-making dilemma. "Others first," once and for all. Or "me first" from now on. Or "work first" come hell or high water. The conflict would then be minimized, but in the process you'd lose the balance.

Unhealthy balance patterns

As you struggle to find the healthy balance pattern for yourself, pay attention to the underlying values, beliefs, and internal messages that guide your balancing choices. You may recognize one of the three unhealthy patterns that most frequently keep people off balance.

Self-absorption

It is possible to get so caught up in your own self-care that you become self-centered, preoccupied, and rigid in your adherence to the "perfect" lifestyle that makes you feel good. "Runners high" is not necessarily a healthy experience.

People who get hooked on taking care of themselves in order to feel good about themselves have little time or inclination for reaching out to others. The trouble with this excessive attention to self-care is that it may end up taking so much focus and energy that there's not much left for building relationships, for showing compassion, or for investing yourself in meaningful work.

Other-absorption

Care-givers are admirable people. They usually have their antennae turned outwards toward others and whenever they pick up signals of need, they are prompted to respond, to reach out—to start caring.

Care giving is extremely fulfilling. It's rewarding to be sensitive, warm, loving, and involved in others' lives. It also feels wonderful to be recognized as a special, caring, loving person.

In fact, helping feels so satisfying that it's possible to get hooked on the experience, becoming addicted to the payoffs of putting others' needs first. The admirable quality of caring for others bears the risk of learning to shortchange yourself—over a long period of time.

Hooked helpers know how to turn their compassion faucet "on" so their love flows out, but they have forgotten how to turn the faucet "off." Addicted care-givers are particularly vulnerable to stress exhaustion. When helpers spend months and even years caring for a parade of "others" without also caring for themselves, they may burn out—and end up feeling empty and bitter.

Overwork

Work is important. Accomplishments and successes breed confidence and allow you to contribute in a positive manner to your world. Those who work hard and take their responsibilities seriously usually are rewarded for their efforts with both praise and promotions. Our culture admires people who produce—and for good reason!

However, hard work and success can become addictive. For work addicts, personal worth becomes dependent upon how much they get done and how successful they become. Fearing failure, addicts soon become driven to succeed. They feel compelled to move from one success to the next, faster and faster.

People who adopt this harried pace create for themselves a life full of distress. They accelerate their tempo—trying to do more and more in less time. They push themselves to accumulate possessions and status; they continually compete with others and with themselves.

The results?—energetic, strong-willed people, independent, capable people, try to achieve greater success, hope to complete all dreams, go faster and faster, and neglect the poetic and personal sides of their lives. These people are caught in a self-made "trap" of attempting to hold everything together, and, one day, are confronted with the question, "Has it been worth the price?"

They awaken to well-earned heart disease or ulcers, to extra-marital affairs, to children gone delinquent, to cold-hearted dismissal from the company to which they "sold" their lives. They are victims of an enlarged sense of duty gone haywire.

Beliefs can trap you

All of us are vulnerable to one or more of these addictive imbalances as we struggle to manage the complexity of our lives and the demands we perceive from self, work, family, and neighbors.

Self-absorption, other-absorption, and overwork usually develop when specific irrational beliefs we hold dear go unchallenged. What about you? What beliefs are likely to trap you in one of these unhealthy patterns?

Use the worksheet below to take a look at the beliefs which underlie each unhealthy imbalance and ask yourself, based on your beliefs, which imbalance pattern is most likely to trap you.

Unhealthy Balance Patterns

■ Read through the list of beliefs underlying the three unhealthy balance patterns below. Remember, these are **unspoken** assumptions—few of us would really say these embarrassing statements out loud! Mark the beliefs in each area that sound similar to some of your own. Check all that apply to you. How many of these assumptions do you whisper to yourself?

Self-absorption

It's a cruel world. Others are only interested in themselves. If I don't take care of myself who will?

I don't have the limits of normal people.

I don't have the obligations of other people.

I am really the center of my life.

Getting what I need, and feeling good about it is the key issue in life.

If I take good care of myself, I can control my life and I won't have to experience much pain.

Maybe I can live forever!

Other-absorption

My needs aren't as important as yours.

It's selfish to take care of myself.

I must be a super helper, able to help everyone, anytime.

I must always try to help someone if I'm asked.

Alhough I feel empty, I can always go to the bottom of the pot and find more to give.

I'll get my needs met after I'm done helping you meet yours.

Overwork

I must always be competent (read "perfect!")

I must always get everything done that I said I would—and on time.

I must work harder than others.

I'm worth more when I work—when I accomplish something I feel more worthwhile.

No matter how capable I am I could have done better.

I'm tough—I can tolerate pain, I don't need much sleep and I can pay whatever price is necessary to get the job done.

■ To which trap are you most vulnerable? _____

_____

■ In what ways have you noticed that the beliefs you whisper to yourself lead you into making choices that cause you distress? _____

_____

■ How could you alter, or at least counter, some of your most troublesome beliefs?

_____

Tips for the self-absorbed

Here are five tips on how to rebalance if you're too absorbed in your own self-care:

Remember that you can't control what happens to you. Try to relax a bit. Don't take yourself so seriously. You may get sick, you may be injured in an accident, or an important relationship may end—and all the self care you can muster up won't do anything to save you from the pain. And in the end you will surely die anyway. So, why not focus on someone other than just you? Why not try to do some good while you're here!

Find people in need and care for them. You don't have to look far to find needy people. So what if you don't know them, or don't like them, or they're not "your type." For what you need to learn about reaching out to others these people will teach you the most.

Make a long term commitment to someone. Stick with your commitment to them no matter how they behave, and no matter how you feel. Commitment is a decision to reach out beyond yourself at a cost and a risk. It is not a feeling!

Attach yourself to a cause you can really believe in. Then use all the skills and resources that you have at your disposal to make your "mission" become a reality.

Attend several funerals. You should be able to find a funeral nearby almost any day! It doesn't matter whether or not you knew the deceased. Sit in the service and think about what is truly important, and valuable, and permanent.

Tips for the hooked care giver

Tips for how to rebalance if you're trying to reach out and care for too many people at once.

Learn to put your own name on the care-giving list. It's great to "Love your neighbor as yourself"; but if you don't take care of yourself you won't have the physical or emotional resources to help your neighbor.

If you're in a real pinch and you don't want to respond to someone else's need, admit that you're a member of "Helper's Anonymous." Say, "I'd like to—but you see, I'm a recovering care-giver and I'm not allowed to help anyone right now!"

Cultivate assertiveness skills. Saying "no" when you need to say "no" and "yes" when you need to say "yes," is essential to recovery.

Don't give up the dream of being a care-giver. It is this very dream that energizes you to reach out to others. Just don't expect to turn your dream into reality 100% of the time, or you'll soon become frustrated and emotionally exhausted.

Determine who most needs your care right now. List their names, and for now, choose to focus care on those people only. Let others wait until later.

Tips for the workaholic

Tips for how to rebalance when you're caught up in too much work and too many outside commitments.

Be honest with yourself. The first step in curing any addiction is an honest self-appraisal. Take a look at yourself. Every person suffers from feelings of insecurity. The workaholic pattern for dealing with these feelings is to prove oneself by working harder and faster. Do you need achievements in order to feel worthwhile? What insecurity are you hiding behind all your racing around? Can you find other methods for becoming lovable?

Evaluate your life. Answer the question, "If I had only one more month to live, what would I do?" Start doing it today! Stop now and make that phone call, write that letter, cry if you need to, forgive someone—whatever you need to do—do it now.

Retrieve your whole personality. Attend to your personal as well as your professional goals. Re-humanize yourself. Concentrate on being a person first. Renew your interest in people. Study faces and learn to love the asymmetry in them. Learn to dream, play, laugh, fantasize, rekindle your curiosity.

Learn to see beauty in the small and the weak. Don't continue to be seduced by size and power; concentrate on appreciating the small and the weak. Take a vacation in your own community. Let the mentally retarded, the chronically ill, the ugly, the sick, or the very old teach you about matters of the heart. They will accept you for who you are. But be forewarned, they probably won't be terribly impressed by your achievements.

Learn that life is unfinished. Nothing is ever fully completed. To be finished is to be dead. Tell yourself, "I won't finish everything today—and that's okay!" Practice leaving partially completed work on your desk. Remember, life is a journey, not a destination.

Recognize your limits

It's tough to make healthy balance decisions because life presents us with more options than we can pursue. It's easy to get caught in the illusion that we can take care of all the needs of others while fully caring for our own at the same time. We can't. The limits of our time and energy force us to compromise, to make choices.

Few people in previous generations expected that all of life's options would be open to them. They weren't tempted to try to keep all their doors open. They tended to accept their "lot in life" and make the best of it. They made choices and got on with their lives.

What makes the healthy balance so difficult to attain for those of our generation is that we've been led to expect that we **can** have it all. We've been seduced into believing that we can do anything that we'd like—maybe even everything!

Well, we can't! And deluding ourselves with the idea that we can keeps us from accepting our limits and making clear choices.

The result? We don't force ourselves to set priorities based on what we value as most important, and we don't activate those values by making clear commitments. We end up spending ourselves in a frenzy, trying to pack into our lives as much as we can, rather than choosing to spend ourselves where we can make the most difference—spending ourselves where we can really count the most.

You alone can decide what to do with your time and energy, but you cannot respond to every opportunity. Your choices to spend yourself are forced choices. When you spend yourself in one way, you necessarily must neglect other options.

You have time to do exactly what you choose to do. You can't make more time. You can't squeeze more into the existing time. You can't save time. You can only spend it—in more or less healthy patterns.

Before moving on to the three-step re-balancing process in the next chapter, stop and reflect on your balance patterns.

Personal Reflection on My Balance Patterns

■ How am I most likely to get myself out of balance? _____

_____

■ Which of my beliefs and my limits must I recognize and adjust before I'll be able to regain my balance?_____

_____

■ What strategy would help me get myself back into a healthy balance? _____

_____

Wish list for my healthy balance

■ List here all your desires and hopes for regaining and maintaining your healthy balance. What would you like to increase? To decrease? To change? Don't limit yourself in any way. The wishes don't have to be practiced.

I wish I could: _____

_____

_____

_____

_____

_____

13

BALANCING
with CLARITY

**A three-step planning guide
to help you gain
and maintain
your healthy balance**

What should you do if you find that your life is currently out of balance and that you are not spending yourself where it counts the most?

Here's a sample three-step planning guide that you can use for yourself whenever you feel the need to try to get yourself back into a balance that's more healthy for you. Memorize these simple steps and use them as needed.

Step 1:
clarify your values

The only way you can spend your time and energy wisely is to know clearly the goals and purposes for which you live and then to make your decisions accordingly.

If your purpose in life is to prove that you can make it on your own, your investment choices will be quite different from someone whose purpose in life is to please others. Your decisions will also be different from those of a person who aims to bring about world peace. If you are deeply committed in your faith, your behavior will reflect your beliefs. If you don't know what you believe or where you're headed in life, you're likely to squander your time and energy resources without making clear choices.

Unfortunately, most of us are only vaguely aware of the beliefs and goals that guide our decision making. In times of great crisis or pain such deeply rooted values come into sharp focus. Priorities suddenly become clear. We know for sure what's important in life and what's worth spending our time and energy on. It's difficult to feel the same clarity of goals and certainty of purpose in the humdrum and hustle-bustle of daily decisions. Yet the same wisdom and spiritual depth must guide these decisions as well.

You don't have to wait for tragedy or death to illuminate your life and point the way to healthy choices. You can use the

worksheet below to help you get in touch with your deepest life
purposes, and then proceed to live out your answers.

Purpose in Life Reflection

- Is it appropriate for you to die? _____

    Why or why not? _____

    When is it appropriate to die? _____

    At what age do you think it would be most appropriate for you to die? _____

    How many years do you have left before you reach that age? _____

- Now focus on the time that is still left. _____

    Ask yourself: Why not die now? _____

    _____

    What's left undone that you should do or be in the remaining time? _____

    _____

    _____

    What should you do with your remaining time so that when you reach your selected age, it
    will be appropriate for you to die—and you can look back over your life with no regrets?

    _____

    _____

- In answering these questions, you've begun to state your purpose in life. What's your sense
    of what you're discovering?

    My life purpose is: _____

    _____

    _____

Step 2:

set healthy balance goals

Gaining and maintaining clarity of purpose and direction will free you to make adjustments in your time- and energy-spending patterns. In light of your internal wisdom about what's most important to you, how would you like to rebalance the various aspects of your life? The worksheet below will help you identify your healthy balance goals.

Healthy Balance Goals

■ Use the circle at the right to illustrate your healthy balance goals. From your current viewpoint, how would you like your circle divided? What would you consider to be the healthiest balance for you? First, indicate your desired **self-care**, **other-care**, and **work** investment balance. Then divide the self-care section into **physical**, **mental**, **relational**, and **spiritual** slices. Divide the **work** investment segment and the **other-care** segment to reflect your desired commitments.

■ Compare your **ideal** healthy balance circle to the one that represents your **current** balance which you drew in Chapter 1.

■ What portions of the circle did you leave the same, indicating that no change is desired?

■ Congratulate yourself for those areas where you feel your investments are already healthy. Affirm for yourself that you're on the right track.

■ What portions of the circle did you change or adjust? Explain why. _____

_____

_____

■ Which areas of the healthy balance do you most need to work on?

self-care _____

other-care _____

work _____

■ What general observations can you now make about your personal priorities and about your current healthy balance level?

I am: _____

_____

_____

■ Summarize the major adjustments in priorities you believe would be healthy for you over the long run.

I'd like to: _____

_____

_____

■ These could be used as your goals for change. Once you're clear about the specific adjustments you'd like to make in your own healthy balance, go back and read the relevant chapter(s) in this book, paying particular attention to the suggestions for change. Then try out some new involvements and see how they work for you.

Step 3:
rebalance regularly

There are no absolute right answers. This is not a recipe book. No one can tell you exactly how to mix the ingredients to bring out the flavor you wish for your life. This book has outlined the resources and principles for obtaining maximum health and wholeness, but the combinations will be your own unique approach. Your personal priorities may indicate that, for you, all aspects of health should not be balanced in equal proportions. Keep on testing until you find the balance that works well for you. Over the years you'll keep adjusting and revising until you find a style that brings you the quality of life that you seek.

You don't have to be perfect. In the preceding chapters you have explored many ideas about physical, mental, relational, and spiritual self-care; about reaching out to family, spouse, and neighbors; about investing yourself in work and in wider issues. Don't try to tackle all of these agendas at once. Remember, the goal is balance, and every change you make, no matter how small, can alter the balance in a healthy direction.

You can tolerate minor imbalance. In fact, perfect adjustment is never possible. Life is unfair. It throws curves, and you will, at times, lurch off balance. You may experience pain, anger, and loneliness. But the tension of imbalance is tolerable, and it will teach you what adjustments you need to make next to regain your balance.

Occasionally you may even purposefully choose to create imbalance. For example, you might stretch your physical limits and go without sleep for a time. Or you might reach out to others who need you, without an immediate full return. Or you might work day and night on a project until it is done. We all learn to live with reality, imperfection, and compromise. These often create an imbalance. That imbalance won't ruin your health, unless it remains too far out of line for too long a time.

Why do you need to rebalance regularly? Because balance is not a noun. It's never a static condition that we can possess and preserve. Balance is a verb. It's an activity that we engage in over and over again as we make mid-course corrections throughout the process of our lives.

How do you carve out a lifestyle that takes seriously your responsibility to others and to your work, without neglecting yourself? How do you find ways to invest in your own self-development without being seduced into the trap of trying to fulfill all of your own needs? How can you find answers to the healthy balance questions?

There are few easy answers and lots of hard questions.

So, get as clear as you can about what's important to you. Then move ahead boldly, making decisions with faith in the future and confidence in your ability to rebalance as necessary.

ADDITIONAL RESOURCES

Seeking Your Healthy Balance is designed as a "workshop-in-a-book"—a hands on tool that can be used for in-depth personal reflection or as a text for participatory classroom instruction and personal support groups. Ultimately, the benefit of this book will be determined solely by the assistance it gives you in finding your healthy balance.

This section offers you suggestions for using **Seeking Your Healthy Balance** most effectively.

Tips for journaling

Tips for use in a discussion group

Thought Provokers
for individual reflection
or group discussion

Tips for journaling

Over time your healthy balance issues will change. So, after you've read this book and completed the worksheets, why not start a journal for keeping track of the ups and downs of your continued search for a healthy balance. Use your journal to record your insights and resolutions for maintaining your balance.

- Start by finding a journal book that feels comfortable to you.
- A journal is not a diary. You don't have to write every day. Just pick up your journal once in a while and write down a few reflections. It's that simple.
- When strong feelings or clear insights come to your mind; tears, laughter, or excitement may well up in you. Terrific! You're in touch with something important. See if you can capture that feeling in words. Be honest with yourself as you write.
- Don't worry about spelling or sentence structure, simply go with the flow of your thoughts. Just get your pen moving across the page, recording the images that come to your mind. Then, see what you discover in the process.
- Use different colored markers to highlight special feelings, to doodle, or to get yourself unstuck.
- Combine music with your journaling. It will help you to slow down and become aware of the emotions and images that may be buried beneath the noise of your hectic schedule.

Record your balance issues

If you develop the habit of regularly recording your own answers to the healthy balance questions, you will find that your journal will become useful to you in a number of ways:

- The process of writing will help you clarify your thinking and feeling about an issue. Writing gives you the opportunity to "talk to yourself" without being heard. You will discover new insights about yourself as you write.

- After you have used your journal for a period of time, you can take the time to read a sampling of your previous entries. You will notice that some themes and patterns occur over and over again in your writing. You may want to pay particular attention to these recurring issues, since they indicate areas which continue to give you trouble. Take note of them. They are important to you and to your life.

- Over the years you will find that some of the more difficult dilemmas you previously wrote about regularly no longer occur as frequently, or not at all. This will give you evidence of the subtle ways in which you have grown and changed.

Why is this so important? Because balance is a verb, not a noun. It's something you keep on doing naturally day after day. You can track this process by keeping a journal of observations about your experiences. Over the years this journal will become a mirror for you, and will teach you the lessons that you most need to know.

Tips for a discussion group

The unique format of **Seeking Your Healthy Balance** is ready-made for discussion groups. It makes your job as a leader easy. The following tips will help you utilize this book most effectively within a small group setting.

Prepare yourself

Here's how to get started.

- Use one chapter as the focus for each session's discussion.
- Answer for yourself all the reader-involvement questions on worksheets in the text.
- Try out the Thought Provokers provided for the chapter and select the one that you think will be most appealing to your group.
- Then, plan the session based on your interests and insights.

The discussion guidelines

Here's what to keep in mind as you listen and share with each other.

When Listening:

- Listen to more than the facts. Try to understand others' experiences and feelings
- Withhold judgment and advice. Encourage others to share their thoughts and feelings, but don't pry or prod, argue or debate.
- Check back with the sharer until he or she feels you understand.

When Sharing:

- Be honest with yourself first. Attend carefully to your experience and feelings, then share what you discover.

- Be specific and precise. Use the pronoun "I." Tell details about yourself—don't talk about "things in general."
- Aim your sharing at the whole group, not just one person.
- Be confident! Others will listen to your story and try to understand.

The discussion process

Here's a suggested outline for the flow of each session.

- Check in with each other. Go around the circle, asking each person to share a short initial reaction to the chapter and how it applied to him or her. This is an important step, but keep it short—more will come later. (10–15 min)
- Discuss any issues that call for deeper sharing or more thorough analysis. Compare answers to the questions in the chapter. Pick up on similarities and differences in themes expressed by the group. Remember, there are no right answers. (10–20 min)
- Explore the topic in more detail by working through the selected Thought Provoker. Take your time and really listen to each other. (30–40 min)
- Check out by going around the group and sharing what the session has meant to you. Comment on yourself and your feelings only, not on the participation of others. After everyone has had a chance to speak, clarify the time and place for the next meeting. (10–15 min)
- Celebrate together. Take a few minutes for an affirmation ritual. (5–10 min)

Thought provokers

This section includes several creative, thought-provoking exercises for each chapter. You can grapple with these questions in your journal, or use them as discussion starters with your family or an established study group. Better yet, why not gather a group of people just for the purpose of sharing and learning together about your individual journeys toward well-being?

Chapter 1   THE HEALTHY BALANCE: Juggling work, self, and others

1. Stop for a moment and reflect on the quality of your life. Are you feeling satisfied? Challenged? At peace? Proud? Energetic? Healthy? Do you have what you want to have?

    Overall, would you agree that you have a good life? Probably your answer is not an unqualified "yes" or "no." We humans are too complicated for easy answers.

    What are the current signs in your life that indicate "yes"—your life is rich, full, and healthy?

    What are the current signs in your life that indicate "no"—your life isn't as healthy as you might wish?

    Share your answers with your family or your group.

2. Look back to pages 7–8 and reflect on the balance between self-care, caring for others, and working that exists in your life right now.

    How much of each focus do you include?

    Has the ratio between self-care, other-care, and work changed for you over the years? How?

    What ratio between these competing responsibilities did you see your parents develop? How do/did you feel about that?

    What ratio would you hope that your children demonstrate?

3. Imagine that you are writing this book.

> Reread the examples of Jeff, Sue, Karl, Carol, and Peggy in this chapter.

> Then write your own healthy balance story, and the stories of your family and friends.

> Read them aloud to each other.

KEEPING BODY and SOUL TOGETHER: Creative self-care   **Chapter 2**

1. Where did you get your ideas about what health is? Your models for how to live a healthy lifestyle? Your training in self-care attitudes and practices?

> First, make a list of all the phrases and attitudes about health that you picked up from your parents ("An apple a day," or "Put on a hat or you'll catch cold," or "Keep a stiff upper lip").

> Share your list with a friend or someone in your group.

> Then brainstorm together all the advertising slogans you can think of that teach something about self-care: ("You deserve a break today," "Plop, plop, fizz, fizz," "When it's time to relax"). What positive or negative self-care message is communicated by each commercial?

2. Based on your present lifestyle and health habits, what type of health breakdown are you working toward? Physical illness? Mental fatigue or emotional upheaval? Relationship difficulties? Spiritual emptiness?

> What kinds of dis-ease are you least likely to suffer because of your positive health habits? Body? Mind? Relationships? Spirit?

3. Everyone needs some private time to be alone for reflection and renewal. Stop for a few minutes and give yourself time to be quiet. Write notes in response to the following questions:

> In your life right now, whom do you need to get away from?
> What pressures do you need to escape from?
> Where could you go for solitude?

Chapter 2

What do you need once you find that "breathing room"?

What's stopping you from getting away right now?

Share your answers with others in your group. Pay special attention to the variety of "get-away" needs people have and the creative excuses we use to avoid our self-care responsibility.

Chapter 3   BUILDING a HEALTHY BODY: Physical self-care

1. Few people are satisfied with their reflections in a mirror. Although we know "God doesn't make no junk," most of us still wonder if God didn't piece us together out of the spare-parts bin.

   Take inventory of yourself as a physical specimen. Which parts seem to be high-quality, factory originals? Your beautiful eyelashes or bulging biceps? Which seem to be inferior-quality, ill-fitting spare parts? Your problem kidney or heavy thighs?

   Draw a picture of your body.

   Spend some time embellishing your drawing. Highlight the weak parts or trouble spots, the vulnerable areas you try to hide or protect.

   Then use another color or different symbols to present your glories and strong points as well.

   Now draw a picture of the physical ideal you would like to reach with proper self-care.

   What kind of body are you dreaming about?
   What do you want to be able to do with it? To have it do for you?
   What changes will you have to make in order to reach these goals?

   Share your pictures and insights with someone in your family or with your group.

2. Where in your body do you usually store tension? What situations tend to make you most tense? Reflect briefly on your relaxation patterns.

   What activities help you relax?
   What memories or mental images bring you peace and tranquillity?
   Are there any special places where you feel particularly calm? What

music helps soothe you?

How often do you take advantage of these tension tamers?

Try a relaxation experience with your group.

3. Write a letter from your body to yourself. Take a whole page or two. Let your body say all it wants you to hear.

Start by writing: "Dear [your name]."

Then get the ball rolling. What does your body want to say about how you exercise it, what you feed it, how you let it rest, the poisons with which you pollute it?

Read your letters out loud and discuss them together as a group.

A BETTER IDEA: Mental self-care

Chapter 4

1. Alone or with a group, list all the feeling words you can think of. Be sure to get over 100, representing a broad spectrum of emotions.

Come to a consensus of your group's top five favorite emotions and your group's five least favorite feelings. Take care that everyone's opinions receive serious consideration in reaching your consensus.

2. Recall a recent experience where something in your life really went wrong. What were the circumstances? What was supposed to happen? What did happen? Why? What got messed up?

Tell the story of the incident to someone else by setting the situation carefully. Then describe in great detail what happened. Dramatize the scene, exaggerating the feelings and incongruities.

3. Think of someone against whom you're holding a grudge. Remember the person and the incident that led to your broken relationship.

Right now force yourself to write a letter of gratitude toward that person.

Don't be cynical or sarcastic. Express your true appreciation. Be thankful for something and see how it changes your attitude.

If you're in a group, read the letter aloud and talk about your feelings.

Remember, revenge eats you alive—not the other person, but you! Gratitude fills you—perhaps the other person as well, but certainly you!

Chapter 5   FILL ME with LOVE: Relational self-care

1. Play the game, "Poor Lonely Me." The rules of the game are simple. Describe to your group your loneliness, your misery, how much you give to others, how overburdened you are, how alone you are, how you're forgotten, how no one understands or appreciates you. Be as dramatic as possible.

   Try to top everyone else's story. Show clearly how you are much worse off than they are. Convince your group that you are the "poorest, loneliest me" there ever was. (Try to take this seriously. Don't laugh. After all, most of us practice this game regularly—we just don't make it so obvious!)

   After you've finished storytelling, talk about how you felt doing this exercise, and how you feel now.

2. This Mind-Reading Dilemma shows you how foolish it is to hope that others will read your mind and give you what you want without your even asking. It will also help you practice asking for what you want.

   On an index card write down something you want right now from someone in your group or from your whole group ("Get off my back," "Please notice me," "Invite me to play racquetball"). Be specific—specific wants, specific person.

   One by one, everyone in the group should try to guess what you wrote on the card. See how close they do or don't come to predicting what you wanted.

   After all have had a turn to guess, read what's on your card. Next, look at the person(s) named on your want card and say "Will you give me this?"

   Then listen for the answers to your request. The other(s) may say "yes" or "no." That's the risk you take. You may not get what you wanted, but at least you asked clearly.

How do you feel? What did you learn by asking for what you want rather than waiting for someone to read your mind?

3. In Taylor Caldwell's novel **The Listener**, people in pain or despair, people burdened with every type of problem, enter the Listener's room and come out healed. At the end of the story the reader finally enters the room to meet the Listener—and finds only a crucifix.

What would you want to tell the Listener were you to enter that room? Write a dialog of your healing encounter with the Listener.

Read your dialog out loud.

Then burn your notes in a fireplace or ashtray. Watch them disappear in smoke. Give your story up to God—and know that you are accepted, forgiven, and no longer alone.

MAGIC MOMENTS: Spiritual self-care   Chapter 6

1. Review the Five Postures for Spiritual Growth described on page 89. Then answer these questions thoughtfully in writing.

Be quiet. How has the noise of a hectic lifestyle gotten in your way lately? What specific noises have made it difficult for you to hear the small voice within you? What do you think this voice is whispering that you've been missing?

Be open to the spiritual. When have you shut out unexpected or unusual spiritual experiences? What kinds of surprises have you missed? What preconceived notions close you off?

Be inquisitive and curious. If you were to actually search for new forms of spiritual experience, what kinds might be revealing, even though they may not fit your normal style? (Prayer groups? Silence? Alternative worship styles?) What do you think you might learn if you experimented with one of these? What specifically would you be afraid of?

Be receptive to pain and grief. What pain have you tried to block out or ignore? If you listen to it, what do you think it will teach you about your depth? What are you afraid of?

Be playful. When have you been so serious that you missed a chance to celebrate and grow in the spirit? Where did you learn that you should be so serious in spiritual matters? Why do you keep believing this? What do you think you could learn by lightening up a bit and becoming more playful?

2. What vocabulary are you most comfortable using when discussing spiritual self-care? What spiritual vocabulary makes you uncomfortable? Take some time to reflect on your language of spiritual well-being.

   Discuss this issue with your group.

   Try, for five minutes, to talk about your spiritual experiences using a language different from your normal style. How do you feel? What do you learn?

   Find someone whose spiritual vocabulary and understanding is quite different from yours. Discuss the issue of spiritual health with this person, listening closely and trying to understand his or her experience fully.

3. All of us have occasional (or frequent) "miracle experiences" in life—times when whatever occurs has little rational explanation and seems to be due to a power beyond us.

   List one or more miracle experiences from your life. Remember and re-feel their depth. Experience the clarity and enthusiasm again. Thank God for them.

   Choose one of your miracle experiences and describe it to somebody else. Celebrate together.

Chapter 7   PUTTING the PIECES TOGETHER: A wholistic view

1. Share your insights from Your Current Health Status Assessment (page 101) with others close to you.

   Ask them how they would have measured your health in each of the four areas based on what they know about you.

   How can you raise or lower your level of well-being? Do you want to make any changes?

2. Refer back to the worksheets on pages 102, 104, and 106. Describe to others your ranking of the four dimensions of self-care.

> Which aspect of health is most important to you? Least?
> Which symptoms do you attend to? Which do you ignore?
> In which areas of health do you least want symptoms?
> Which area is preferable if you must have symptoms?
> To which area of self-care do you usually go first to find remedies?
> Which least? Or never?

If you're doing this exercise with others, compile a group average ranking. Then compare yourself with the group norm.

> Are your priorities and preferences similar to or different from those of others? What does that say about the potential strengths and weaknesses in your self-care practices?

3. Identify your "health care providers" in each of the dimensions of well-being.

> To whom do you turn for physical care? For your annual mental checkup? For relationship prescriptions? For spiritual diagnosis?

> Which of these resources has the most "wholistic" approach?

Share your responses with your group and discuss together possible strategies for pursuing whole person well-being in your self-care practices and choice of health care providers.

BEING WELL-to-DO: The reach-out dimension

Chapter 8

1. Make a diagram showing your purpose-in-life timeline. Recall the first time you can remember being aware of a purpose outside yourself (wanting to help a blind person cross the street, giving a gift to your mom, bringing canned goods for the food shelf).

> From that point, chart your growth in sense of purpose over the years. What twists and turns has the line taken as you've opened some doors in commitment and closed others in surrender?

> Have there been dry spells? Draw them.

> Label the turning points (confirmation, first job, divorce), the

difficult choices, the changing purposes (draft resistance, right to life), the new investments.

Extend your purpose line into the future, predicting what growth looms ahead for you.

Trade timelines with someone else in your group. After studying the diagram for a few minutes, do your best to introduce that person to the group by describing two of his or her life purposes.

Share your timeline with your parents or someone who knows you very well. Can that person describe your journey from the diagram alone?

2. Summarize and discuss with others the results of your Reach-Out Inventory on pages 118–119.

Listen to their stories and try to become aware of how each person has chosen unique, individual patterns for reaching out.

Can you learn anything from the style of others that prompts you to revise or reaffirm your pattern of outreach commitments?

3. Make a random list of all the people and concerns for which you currently feel responsibility. Include all your worries and everything you're trying to control. Be sure to keep writing until your list includes at least 50 items—100 would be better.

When you stop writing look over the list. Notice how you feel.
Then group the items into categories and prioritize them.
Note your reactions and observations.

Share your discoveries with someone else. See how they respond.

Chapter 9 CARING for YOUR FAMILY: Reach out to the people close to you

1. List some of the spoken and unspoken rules that govern conduct and relationships in your family ("Don't talk about our family with others," "We must always stick together," "Never talk back to your parents").

Have any of these rules changed over the years?
Are the rules the same in your family of choice as they were in your family of origin?

How has your family been affected by these rules?

Which are you convinced are essential?

Which could be modified or dropped?

What happens when someone in the family doesn't follow the rules?

How does your family deal with personal limitations, mistakes, transgressions of rules?

How does your family deal with family problems that involve everyone?

How does your family announce forgiveness to each other?

With your family or group develop a forgiveness/acceptance ritual that you can use during difficult times.

2. Examine the costs and rewards of your marriage commitment. Complete the following sentences:

Because of my commitment to my spouse, I cannot _____ and I probably will never be able to _____ and I choose to _____ in spite of some of my wishes.

Because of my commitment to my spouse, I have received _____. I have experienced rewards I would otherwise never have known such as_____, _____, _____, _____ and _____.

Put yourself in your spouse's shoes and complete the sentences again as you imagine he or she might.

Then spend 15 minutes with your partner, sharing your answers and brainstorming the strengths and rewards of your relationship.

3. Draw a picture of your family with you in it. Use symbols, words, or colors to show the connections between members.

What signs of health and unhealth do you see in your family portrait?

Did you include any member of your extended family in your picture? Why? Why not? How do they, or don't they, fit into your family?

Share your drawing with the rest of the family and discuss ways you all could make an even more healthy investment in each other.

Chapter 10 CARING for OTHERS: Reach out to the people around you

1. Imagine you are in the studio audience at a talk show when the authors of **Seeking Your Healthy Balance** are being interviewed. You are asked to give them feedback about your perception of the benefits of caring for others. What do you say?

   How do you describe your life as a care-giver? What has been the toughest aspect that you've had to deal with? What has been the most freeing? Most rewarding? Most draining?

   Make notes of those issues on which you want to speak your piece.

   Compare you stories, feelings, and insights with others in the studio audience (your group, family, or friends). What common denominators do you find?

2. Hug—or in some other way physically touch—the next three people you speak to. Yes, no matter where you are or who you're with! No matter what the circumstances. Touch them! See what happens. If you're with people you trust, talk about what you just did and share your reactions.

3. Look for signs of human need in the newspaper. Read all the articles, features, ads, classifieds. As you read each, ask yourself, "What is needed here? Who needs my caring? How could I reach out?"

   Make a list of the needs you discover just from creatively reading the paper. Don't stop with less that 100!

   Choose one of these local needs and plan a strategy for reaching out to the person(s). Put your plan into action and report back to your group.

INVESTING in MEANINGFUL WORK: Reach out to your world   # Chapter 11

1. On a blank sheet of paper draw a picture of your work setting and your work organization with yourself in it. You don't need to be an artist. Use symbols, diagrams, words, characterizations—whatever you like.

   Examine your picture and embelish it. Symbolize in your picture all the ways in which you reach out responsibly in your job attempting to make a positive difference.

   Then, symbolize in your picture all the personal benefits you gain from your job—the elements of your work that nurture you.

   Examine what you have drawn and make at least three summary observations about what you see (or don't see) in your picture.

   Share your picture and your insights with someone else.

2. Write down the name of a person who reaches out to his or her world as an unsung hero or heroine. It could be a person you've only read about (Florence Nightingale, Martin Luther King, Mahatma Gandhi), or someone as caring and principled from your own private circle.

   Meditate on the qualities of this person for five minutes; then answer these questions:

   What is his character? Her focus? What makes him or her so special? So admirable?

   In what ways would you like to emulate this person—in your work and your service? What would be a first step you could take?

   Compare heroes and heroines with others in your group. Then for the next week, take a poll on unsung heroes and heroines. Ask everyone you meet about his or hers. Keep track of all the suggestions and report back to your group.

3. Make a list of what you consider to be the moral issues of your time—include international, national, state, and local issues. Then ask yourself what you are doing to respond to each in a manner that fits your beliefs and priorities.

Chapter 12 RECOGNIZING UNHEALTHY PATTERNS:
The healthy balance revisited

1. Reconsider the three unhealthy balance patterns identified in this chapter—self-absorption, other-absorption, and overwork.

   Write an essay to yourself about the ways in which you are most likely to get yourself out of balance, the beliefs that consistently erode your balance, and the effect that this pattern has on your personal well-being.

   Share your essay with someone else.

   Write out your personal dialog in response to these questions:

   Do you have a right to take care of yourself?
   Do you have a responsibility to take care of yourself?
   "Yes," because . . . . "No," because . . . .

   Pair up with someone and read your list together and put it on a blackboard or newsprint.

   Talk about the process and your personal dialogs.

   How do you decide when to care for you and when to care for others? What's your typical pattern? How often do you decide one way or the other?

   In what specific situations do you always say "no" or always say "yes"?

2. If you have been using the Thought Provokers chapter-by-chapter in a discussion group, you might like to complete the experience with the following closure exercise.

   Make a health report card for each person in your discussion group.

   Use an index card for each person.
   List the three positive health habits you admire in that person (optimistic attitude, service in the community, intensity of feeling, empathy, etc.).

   Then go around the group telling each person directly the qualities you appreciate, giving specific examples of healthy behavior you have observed.

After each person has given and received appreciation from every member, sign each person's report card and give it to him or her with a wish for continued well-being.

BALANCING with CLARITY: A three-step planning process   **Chapter 13**

1. Write a brief eulogy for yourself, as if you had lived out your answers to the Purpose in Life Reflection (page 179). How would you like to be remembered?

   As a group, take turns reading your eulogies out loud.

2. Share your Healthy Balance Goals (page 180) with your group or a significant other.

   Set a date and time to get together again six months or a year from now to compare notes on your healthy balance experiences.